PHYSICAL FITNESS LABORATORIES
ON A BUDGET

TERRY J. HOUSH
University of Nebraska–Lincoln

JOEL T. CRAMER
University of Oklahoma

JOSEPH P. WEIR
Des Moines University

TRAVIS W. BECK
University of Oklahoma

GLEN O. JOHNSON
University of Nebraska–Lincoln

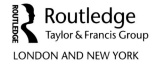

LONDON AND NEW YORK

Library of Congress Cataloging-in-Publication Data

Physical fitness laboratories on a budget / Terry Housh ... [et al.].
    p. ; cm.
  Includes bibliographical references and index.
  ISBN 978-1-890871-90-1
1. Physical fitness--Testing. 2. Exercise--Physiological aspects. 3. Exercise tests. I. Housh,
Terry J. [DNLM: 1. Physical Fitness—physiology—Laboratory Manuals. 2. Exercise Test—
methods—Laboratory Manuals. QT 25 P578 2009]
  QP301.P558 2009
  612.7'6—dc22

                                                        2008029522

First published 2009 by Holcomb Hathaway, Publishers, Inc.

Published 2017 by Routledge
2 Park Square, Milton Park, Abingdon, Oxfordshire OX14 4RN
711 Third Avenue, New York, NY 10017, USA

First issued in hardback 2017

Routledge is an imprint of the Taylor & Francis Group, an informa business

ISBN 13: 978-1-138-07836-9 (hbk)
ISBN 13: 978-1-890871-90-1 (pbk)

Contents

ver the past several decades, we have seen a dramatic increase in interest in physical fitness as it relates to health and sports performance. As a result, the number of academic programs that train professionals in the various scientific aspects of exercise and sport science, as well as healthy lifestyles, has also increased. These programs are designed to prepare students for careers in physical activity settings such as YMCAs/YWCAs, health clubs, and corporate fitness centers, as well as public and private schools, where a health and fitness orientation is becoming commonplace in physical education and health classes. Often, college and university courses in physical fitness, exercise physiology, and healthy lifestyles include not only classroom work, but also laboratory and active learning experiences. Many institutions of higher education, however, do not have the equipment, facilities, and/or budget to provide students with high-tech laboratory experiences. *Physical Fitness Laboratories on a Budget* provides meaningful laboratory experiences that can be taught without sophisticated and expensive equipment. The most expensive piece of equipment needed for the laboratories in this text is a cycle ergometer, and many of the laboratories require little or no equipment.

This text is designed for physical fitness, exercise physiology, and healthy lifestyles courses, among others, and covers seven major components of physical fitness: aerobic fitness, fatigue thresholds, muscular strength, muscular endurance, muscular power, body composition and body build, and flexibility. Laboratories include the following sections: Background, Terms and Abbreviations, Equipment (and pricing), Procedures, Equations, Sample Calculations, Worksheets, Tables, Extension Activities, Extension Questions, and References.

The Background section of each lab provides students with the information they'll need to understand what will be measured in the laboratory. The Terms and Abbreviations checklist familiarizes readers with the language and symbols used throughout the lab. The list of equipment corresponds to the list of vendors for such equipment in Appendix 2, to assist students and instructors in finding the most cost-effective equipment available. The Procedures sections, which contain step-by-step directions, are clear and logical with photographic examples to guide students through the various parts of the lab. Equations and sample calculations vital to the laboratory are included. Many of the laboratories in this text involve the application of mathematical modeling to physiological systems. This allows instructors and students the opportunity to apply basic mathematics, statistical analyses, and computer applications to discussions of how the systems of the body work. Lab Worksheets allow students to perform the given lab using either themselves or classmates as subjects and to record their responses. The Extension Activities and Questions sections provide students additional opportunities to practice the lab procedures and explore issues of validity, reliability, and accuracy related to them.

The authors of this text have a common association through the University of Nebraska–Lincoln. Over the years, these associations have grown into close friendships, making the opportunity to coauthor this text a true personal and professional pleasure. Dr. Glen O. Johnson (along with Dr. William G. Thorland) began the Ph.D. program in Exercise Physiology at UNL in the late 1970s. Dr. Johnson served as a mentor to the other coauthors of this manual, and Dr. Terry J. Housh was the first Ph.D. graduate in 1984. Drs. Joseph P. Weir, Joel T. Cramer, and Travis W. Beck received Ph.D. degrees in 1993, 2003, and 2007, respectively. Today, Drs. Johnson and Housh are professors in the Department of Nutrition and Health Sciences at UNL and continue to advise Exercise Physiology doctoral students. Dr. Weir is a professor in the Doctor of Physical Therapy Program at Des Moines University Osteopathic Medical Center, where he supervises the research of Physical Therapy students. Drs. Cramer and Beck are assistant professors in the Department of Health and Exercise Science at the University of Oklahoma, where they mentor Exercise Physiology Ph.D. students.

In addition to this manual, the authors worked together on the text *Introduction to Exercise Science* (Holcomb Hathaway, 2008) with Terry Housh and Glen Johnson as authors and editors. Joel Cramer and Travis Beck contributed the chapters Reading and Interpreting the Literature in Exercise Science, and Exercise Epidemiology. Joseph Weir contributed the Exercise Physiology chapter. Terry Housh is also author of *Applied Exercise and Sport Physiology,* Second Edition (Holcomb Hathaway, 2006).

Acknowledgments

Our sincere thanks to the following reviewers of the manuscript, who offered constructive ideas for improving the manual: Lisa Augustine, Lorraine Community College; Shane Callahan, Lewis and Clark Community College; Mandi Dupain, Millersville University, Pennsylvania; Joan M. Eckerson, Creighton University; Tammy K. Evetovich, Wayne State College; Sara A. Glover, Loras College; Doug Herndon, Lorain County Community College; Tom Hood, Doane College; Patricia Jensen, York College of Nebraska; Paul McDonough, University of Texas at Arlington; John McLester, Kennesaw State University; Kathy Tritschler, Guilford College; and Judy Wilson, University of Texas at Arlington.

We would also like to acknowledge doctoral students Michelle Mielke, Clayton Camic, C. Russell Hendrix, and Jorge Zuniga of the University of Nebraska–Lincoln for their assistance during the writing of this manual.

Unit 1

INTRODUCTION

1

BACKGROUND

The American College of Sports Medicine (ACSM) recommends that medical supervision is not necessary during exercise for healthy individuals (children, adolescents, men <45 years of age, and women <55 years of age) who have no symptoms or known presence of heart disease or major coronary risk factors.[1] Therefore, the primary purpose of preparticipation health screening is to identify those individuals who should be excluded from exercise due to medical contraindications.

The ACSM has provided recommendations for preparticipation health screening procedures for various populations.[1] Specifically, the ACSM defines preparticipation health screening as a three-step process that involves: (a) risk stratification and medical clearance, (b) additional preparticipation assessment, and (c) exercise test considerations. Of these three steps, risk stratification and medical clearance are the most important for performing exercise testing with healthy individuals. Additional preparticipation assessment and exercise test considerations are necessary when evaluating the elderly and individuals with disease conditions that could limit their ability to perform physical activity.

In addition, it may be important to have potential participants complete an informed consent document. The primary purpose of the informed consent document is to provide potential participants with clear and exact information about what they will be required to do during the exercise test. When participants fully understand what they must do, they will be instructed to sign the informed consent document, after which they will be allowed to do the exercise test. Page 4 shows an example of an informed consent document for a maximum one-repetition bench press (1-RM strength test).

With the exception of clinical exercise physiology laboratories and cardiac rehabilitation centers, most exercise science laboratories examine normal, healthy individuals. However, some individuals may not be aware of their risk stratification, so it is essential that careful screening procedures be completed. If the results of a preparticipation health screening questionnaire indicate that an individual may be at a health risk for exercise, the individual should be encouraged to obtain medical clearance before participation. Determination of whether an individual is actually at risk for exercise can, however, be vague. Thus, the purpose of this laboratory is to describe the procedures used to perform preparticipation health screening.

KNOW THESE TERMS & ABBREVIATIONS

- ☐ ACSM = American College of Sports Medicine
- ☐ 1-RM = one-repetition maximum
- ☐ PAR-Q = Physical Activity Readiness Questionnaire
- ☐ risk stratification = categorization of the likelihood of untoward events based on the screening and evaluation of patient health characteristics

EQUIPMENT

N/A

Approximate Price

N/A

PROCEDURES

(See photo 1.1.) An individual's risk during exercise can be assessed with a medical screening instrument such as the Physical Activity Readiness Questionnaire (PAR-Q; see page 5) or a Pre-exercise Testing Health Status Questionnaire (see pages 6–7). The PAR-Q is a common medical screening instrument used by many exercise physiology laboratories. The procedures used to determine risk stratification from both the PAR-Q and Pre-exercise Testing Health Status Questionnaire are described below.

PAR-Q

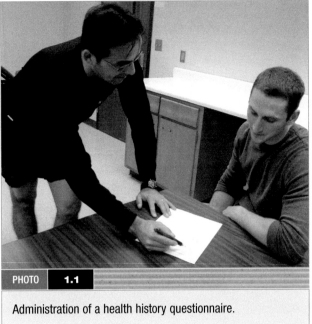

PHOTO **1.1**

Administration of a health history questionnaire.

1. Begin administering the PAR-Q by instructing the individual to complete the first seven questions.
2. If the individual answers "yes" to one or more of the first seven questions, instruct him or her to contact a physician before performing any exercise. Inform the individual that he or she should tell the physician which questions had "yes" answers on the PAR-Q. The individual should also ask the physician what exercise tests should or should not be performed.
3. If the individual answers "no" to all of the first seven questions, he or she should be allowed to perform the exercise test.

Pre-exercise Testing Health Status Questionnaire

1. Begin the Pre-exercise Testing Health Status Questionnaire by instructing the individual to complete the general information at the top of the questionnaire and sections A through G.
2. Examine the completed questionnaire and determine whether the individual can safely perform the exercise test that you are asking him or her to do. If you feel that the individual may be at a health risk during the exercise test, instruct him or her to contact a physician and receive medical clearance before performing the test.

REFERENCE

1. American College of Sports Medicine. *ACSM's Guidelines for Exercise Testing and Prescription,* 7th edition. Philadelphia: Lippincott Williams & Wilkins, 2006.

INFORMED CONSENT FOR A BENCH PRESS 1-RM TEST

1. Purpose and Explanation of the Test

You will perform a one-repetition maximum (1-RM) bench press strength test using an Olympic barbell, weight plates, and a standard free weight bench. To begin the test, you will perform a warm-up with just the barbell. For each warm-up repetition, you will be required to lower the weight to your chest and then press it upward until your forearms are fully extended. Following the warm-up repetitions, additional weight will be added to the bar, and you will be asked to perform one repetition. If you can successfully complete the repetition, you will be allowed to rest for two minutes while additional weights are added to the bar. You will then be asked to perform one repetition with the new weight. Weights will be continually added to the bar until you are no longer able to complete the movement throughout the full range of motion. The heaviest weight that you were able to lift once will be your bench press 1-RM.

2. Attendant Risks and Discomforts

There is a slight possibility of straining or tearing a muscle during the bench press 1-RM test. Elevations in blood pressure and lightheadedness immediately after the strength test may occur. You may experience muscle soreness for a few days after the test. Every effort will be made to minimize potential risks by allowing for a thorough warm-up prior to the 1-RM test.

3. Responsibilities of the Participant

Information you present about your health status and previous experiences of muscle or joint injuries (e.g., muscle strains, tears, joint dislocations) may affect the safety of your strength test. Your prompt reporting of these conditions is very important to ensure that you are not injured during the 1-RM test. In addition, you will be asked several times during the strength test if you feel any joint or muscle pain.

4. Benefits to Be Expected

The results obtained from your test will provide information regarding your upper-body strength. This information may be helpful for you in the design of future training programs.

5. Inquiries

You are encouraged to ask any questions about the procedures used in the exercise test or the results of your test. If you have any concerns or questions, please ask us for further explanations.

6. Use of Medical Records

The information that is obtained during exercise testing will be treated as privileged and confidential as described in the Health Insurance Portability and Accountability Act of 1996. It is not to be released or revealed to any person except your referring physician without your written consent. However, the information obtained may be used for statistical analysis or scientific purposes with your right to privacy retained.

7. Freedom of Consent

I hereby consent to engage voluntarily in an exercise test to determine my upper-body strength. My permission to perform this test is given voluntarily. I understand that I am free to stop the test at any point if I so desire.

I have read this form, and I understand the test procedures that I will perform and the attendant risks and discomforts. Knowing these risks and discomforts, and having had an opportunity to ask questions that have been answered to my satisfaction, I consent to participate in this test.

Date 10/16/23   _Signature of Participant_

Date 10/16/23   _Signature of Witness_

Date 10/16/23   _Signature of Person Conducting the Test_

Physical Activity Readiness
Questionnaire - PAR-Q
(revised 2002)

PAR-Q & YOU

(A Questionnaire for People Aged 15 to 69)

Regular physical activity is fun and healthy, and increasingly more people are starting to become more active every day. Being more active is very safe for most people. However, some people should check with their doctor before they start becoming much more physically active.

If you are planning to become much more physically active than you are now, start by answering the seven questions in the box below. If you are between the ages of 15 and 69, the PAR-Q will tell you if you should check with your doctor before you start. If you are over 69 years of age, and you are not used to being very active, check with your doctor.

Common sense is your best guide when you answer these questions. Please read the questions carefully and answer each one honestly: check YES or NO.

YES	NO		
☐	☐	1.	**Has your doctor ever said that you have a heart condition <u>and</u> that you should only do physical activity recommended by a doctor?**
☐	☐	2.	**Do you feel pain in your chest when you do physical activity?**
☐	☐	3.	**In the past month, have you had chest pain when you were not doing physical activity?**
☐	☐	4.	**Do you lose your balance because of dizziness or do you ever lose consciousness?**
☐	☐	5.	**Do you have a bone or joint problem (for example, back, knee or hip) that could be made worse by a change in your physical activity?**
☐	☐	6.	**Is your doctor currently prescribing drugs (for example, water pills) for your blood pressure or heart condition?**
☐	☐	7.	**Do you know of <u>any other reason</u> why you should not do physical activity?**

If

you

answered

YES to one or more questions

Talk with your doctor by phone or in person BEFORE you start becoming much more physically active or BEFORE you have a fitness appraisal. Tell your doctor about the PAR-Q and which questions you answered YES.

- You may be able to do any activity you want — as long as you start slowly and build up gradually. Or, you may need to restrict your activities to those which are safe for you. Talk with your doctor about the kinds of activities you wish to participate in and follow his/her advice.
- Find out which community programs are safe and helpful for you.

NO to all questions

If you answered NO honestly to <u>all</u> PAR-Q questions, you can be reasonably sure that you can:
- start becoming much more physically active — begin slowly and build up gradually. This is the safest and easiest way to go.
- take part in a fitness appraisal — this is an excellent way to determine your basic fitness so that you can plan the best way for you to live actively. It is also highly recommended that you have your blood pressure evaluated. If your reading is over 144/94, talk with your doctor before you start becoming much more physically active.

DELAY BECOMING MUCH MORE ACTIVE:
- if you are not feeling well because of a temporary illness such as a cold or a fever — wait until you feel better; or
- if you are or may be pregnant — talk to your doctor before you start becoming more active.

PLEASE NOTE: If your health changes so that you then answer YES to any of the above questions, tell your fitness or health professional. Ask whether you should change your physical activity plan.

<u>Informed Use of the PAR-Q</u>: The Canadian Society for Exercise Physiology, Health Canada, and their agents assume no liability for persons who undertake physical activity, and if in doubt after completing this questionnaire, consult your doctor prior to physical activity.

No changes permitted. You are encouraged to photocopy the PAR-Q but only if you use the entire form.

NOTE: If the PAR-Q is being given to a person before he or she participates in a physical activity program or a fitness appraisal, this section may be used for legal or administrative purposes.

"I have read, understood and completed this questionnaire. Any questions I had were answered to my full satisfaction."

NAME _____

SIGNATURE _____ DATE_____

SIGNATURE OF PARENT _____ WITNESS _____
or GUARDIAN (for participants under the age of majority)

Note: This physical activity clearance is valid for a maximum of 12 months from the date it is completed and becomes invalid if your condition changes so that you would answer YES to any of the seven questions.

 © Canadian Society for Exercise Physiology   Supported by: 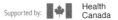 Health   Santé
                                                                              Canada Canada   continued on other side...

PRE-EXERCISE TESTING HEALTH STATUS QUESTIONNAIRE

Name _Mohamed Mages_   Date _10/16/23_

ID# _____   Birthdate (mm/dd/yy) _11/09/2000_

Home Address _____

Work Phone _(806) 363-4458_   Home Phone _N/A_

E-mail Address _mager09@gmail.com_

Person to contact in case of emergency _Hadi Bakate_

Emergency Contact Phone _(806) 324-3251_

Personal Physician _N/A_   Physician's Phone _N/A_

Gender _Male_   Age (yrs) _22_

Height (ft) (in) _5 6_   Weight (lbs) _145_

Does the above weight indicate: ● *a gain* ○ *a loss* ○ *no change* in the past year?
If a change, how many pounds? _____5_____ (lbs)

A. JOINT-MUSCLE STATUS (✔ *Check areas where you currently have problems.*)

JOINT AREAS

○ Wrists   ○ Hips
○ Elbows   ○ Knees
○ Shoulders   ○ Ankles
○ Upper spine & neck   ○ Feet
○ Lower spine   ○ Other

MUSCLE AREAS

○ Arms   ○ Lower back
○ Shoulders   ○ Buttocks
○ Chest   ○ Thighs
○ Upper back & neck   ○ Lower leg
○ Abdominal regions   ○ Feet

B. HEALTH STATUS (✔ *Check if you previously had or currently have any of the following conditions.*)

○ High blood pressure
○ Heart disease or dysfunction
○ Peripheral circulatory disorder
○ Lung disease or dysfunction
○ Arthritis or gout
○ Edema
○ Epilepsy
○ Multiple sclerosis
○ High blood cholesterol or triglyceride levels
○ Loss of consciousness
○ Other conditions that you feel we should
know about _____
_____
_____

○ Pregnant

○ Acute infection
○ Diabetes or blood sugar level abnormality
○ Anemia
○ Hernias
○ Thyroid dysfunction
○ Pancreas dysfunction
○ Liver dysfunction
○ Kidney dysfunction
○ Phenylketonuria (PKU)
○ Allergic reactions to medication
Please describe:
_____
_____

○ Allergic reactions to any other substance
Please describe:
_____

QUESTIONNAIRE, page 2

C. PHYSICAL EXAMINATION HISTORY

Approximate date of your last physical examination _____9 / 13 / 2021_____

Physical problems noted at that time _____None_____

Has a physician ever made any recommendations relative to limiting your level of physical exertion?   YES (NO)

If YES, what limitations were recommended? _____

Have you ever had an abnormal resting electrocardiogram (ECG)?   YES (NO)

D. CURRENT MEDICATION USAGE (List the drug name and the condition being managed.)

MEDICATION   CONDITION

E. PHYSICAL PERCEPTIONS (Indicate any unusual sensations or perceptions. ✔ Check if you have recently experienced any of the following during or soon after physical activity (PA) or during sedentary periods (SED).)

PA	SED		PA	SED	
○	○	Chest pain	○	○	Nausea
○	○	Heart palpitations "fast irregular heartbeats"	○	○	Lightheadedness
○	○	Unusually rapid breathing	○	○	Loss of consciousness
○	○	Overheating	○	○	Loss of balance
○	○	Muscle cramping	○	○	Loss of coordination
○	○	Muscle pain	○	○	Extreme weakness
○	○	Joint pain	○	○	Numbness
○	○	Other	○	○	Mental confusion

F. FAMILY HISTORY (✔ Check if any of your blood relatives—parents, brothers, sisters, aunts, uncles, and/or grandparents—have or had any of the following.)

○ Heart disease

○ Heart attacks or strokes (prior to age 50)

○ Elevated blood cholesterol or triglyceride levels

○ High blood pressure

○ Diabetes

○ Sudden death (other than accidental)

G. CURRENT HABITS (✔ Check any of the following if they are characteristic of your current habits.)

○ Smoking. If so, how many per day? _____

○ Regularly does manual gardening or yardwork.

○ Regularly goes for long walks.

○ Frequently rides a bicycle.

○ Frequently runs/jogs for exercise.

○ Regularly participates in a weight training exercise program.

○ Engages in a sports program more than once per week.

  If so, what does the program consist of?

_____

Worksheet 1.1   EXTENSION ACTIVITIES

Name _____ Date _____

1. Administer the PAR-Q and Pre-exercise Testing Health Status Questionnaire to someone in your class. Based on the results from the questionnaires, could the individual safely perform the following exercise tests? Circle the appropriate answer next to each exercise test.

    (YES)   NO   Bench Press One-Repetition Maximum (1-RM) Strength Test

    (YES)   NO   Leg Extension One-Repetition Maximum (1-RM) Strength Test

    (YES)   NO   Submaximal Cycle Ergometer Test

    (YES)   NO   Maximal Cycle Ergometer Test

    (YES)   NO   Maximal Treadmill Test

    (YES)   NO   Flexibility Test

    (YES)   NO   Test for Anaerobic Power

2. Complete the PAR-Q and Pre-exercise Testing Health Status Questionnaire for yourself. Based on the results, determine whether you would be able to perform most exercise tests safely.

    I will be able to perform all exercises safely

BACKGROUND

Several different physical fitness assessments may involve the measurement of a basic vital sign: heart rate (HR). Sometimes the measurement is performed at rest, which can help determine the pre-exercise health status of the individual or the return to resting conditions after exercise. During exercise, monitoring HR can be an effective method to estimate the intensity of exercise, especially during aerobic exercise. Heart rate is directly related to exercise intensity, and this relationship is most predictable between 50% and 90% of the maximum HR.[1] In addition, for exercise at the same absolute work rate, the HR of an aerobically trained individual will be lower than that of an untrained or unfit person. Thus, for someone who is less physically fit, the HR will generally be higher after completing a fitness test. For example, the Queen's College Step Test (see Lab 6) is based on the assumption that less fit individuals will have a higher HR after the three-minute step test than subjects who are more physically fit. Therefore, measuring HR before, during, and after exercise is an important aspect of physical fitness testing.

On average, most people have resting HR values between 60 and 80 beats per minute (bpm).[4] However, the average resting HR for women tends to be 7–10 bpm higher than for men.[4] Table 2.1 provides specific normative values for resting HR. There are three common clinical classifications of resting HR:

1. Bradycardia, defined as a slow HR of less than 60 bpm
2. Tachycardia, a fast HR of greater than 100 bpm
3. Normal rhythm, a resting HR of 60–100 bpm

Norms for resting heart rate in men and women (age = 18–65+ years). | TABLE 2.1

Classification	Resting heart rate (bpm)	
	MEN	WOMEN
Low	35–56	39–58
Moderately low	57–61	59–63
< Average	62–65	64–67
Average	66–71	68–72
> Average	72–75	73–77
Moderately high	76–81	78–83
High	82–103	84–104

Data from Golding, L. A. (2000). *YMCA fitness testing and assessment manual.* Champaign, IL: Human Kinetics.

Two primary methods are used for assessing resting HR: (a) palpation and (b) a heart rate monitor. The most common and cost-effective method for measuring HR is palpation. A more expensive but convenient method that has become increasingly popular is a digital-display HR monitor. Procedures for both methods are described below.

KNOW THESE TERMS & ABBREVIATIONS

☐ HR = heart rate, measured in beats per minute (bpm)

☐ HR monitor = equipment used to measure and monitor heart rate; includes a chest strap (identifies the heartbeats and transmits the signal telemetrically) and a digital display (displays the signal as a real-time HR value)

☐ palpation = the act of examining by touch

EQUIPMENT (see Appendix 2 for vendors)   **Approximate Price**

1. Stopwatch (photo 2.1) $10
2. Heart rate monitor (photo 2.2) $100

PROCEDURES

Palpation[3]

1. To palpate the HR (or pulse), use the tips of the index and middle fingers. Avoid using the thumb, since small arteries running through the thumb can be confused with the actual palpable HR.

2. Palpate one of the following anatomical landmarks to find the pulse:

   a. The radial artery, which is located on the anterior-lateral surface of the wrist, in line with the base of the thumb.[4] The best location is usually just medial to the styloid process of the radius. The tips of

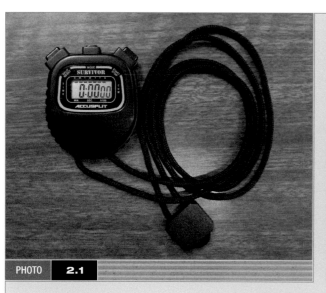

PHOTO **2.1**

A stopwatch.

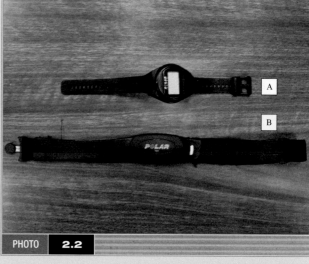

PHOTO **2.2**

A heart rate monitor system: (A) digital display, (B) chest strap.

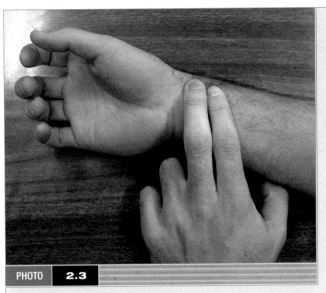

PHOTO   2.3

Palpation of the radial artery pulse.

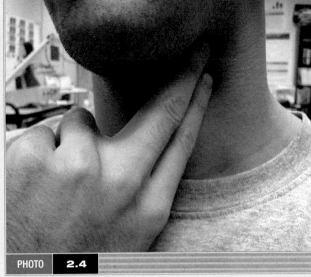

PHOTO   2.4

Palpation of the carotid artery pulse.

the index and middle fingers should be placed gently on the skin over this area (photo 2.3).

b. The carotid artery can be found on the anterior surface of the neck, just lateral to the larynx (photo 2.4).[4] Care should be taken when palpating the pulse of the carotid artery, because applying too much pressure may artificially lower the resultant HR value.[5,8] This may be due to negative feedback from the baroreceptors, which sense pressure, in the aortic arch. There is some debate in the literature whether carotid artery palpation elicits enough pressure to trigger the baroreceptors.[2,6,7]

3. Once the pulse is located, use a stopwatch (photo 2.1) to keep the time while counting the beats. If the stopwatch is started at the moment the counting begins, count the first beat as "0." If the stopwatch has been running, count the first beat as "1."

4. The HR should be counted for a set period of time, such as 10, 15, 30, or 60 seconds. Use one of the following calculations to determine the HR in beats per minute (bpm):

   a. Counting for 10 seconds: Take the number of beats counted and multiply by 6.

   b. Counting for 15 seconds: Take the number of beats counted and multiply by 4.

   c. Counting for 30 seconds: Take the number of beats counted and multiply by 2.

5. Generally, the shorter-duration HR counts (10 and 15 seconds) are used during and after exercise, when it is important to attain a momentary HR. Since HR can increase with exercise intensity and decrease during recovery, it is sometimes necessary to count the beats during short time periods to obtain an accurate representation of HR at a specific moment during exercise or recovery. In contrast, resting HR measurements are often counted for 30 or 60 seconds to reduce the risk of miscounts and error.

Heart Rate Monitor

Generally, a HR monitor consists of a chest strap and a digital display (photo 2.5). The chest strap contains sensors that identify the heartbeats, and the resultant signal is transmitted telemetrically to the digital display as a real-time HR value in bpm. As with all equipment, different HR monitors may function slightly differently, and the manufacturer's directions should be read and followed. However, most HR monitors work in a similar fashion, and the procedure is as follows:

PHOTO 2.5

Placement of the heart rate monitor strap and the digital display of resting heart rate.

1. Most chest straps require a little moisture (water) applied with a damp cloth over the sensor areas to improve their ability to sense heartbeats.

2. Once the chest strap has been wetted, place the strap just distal to the pectoralis major muscles by adjusting the elastic band (see photo 2.5). The strap should be firm, but not tight enough to indent the skin. For both men and women, the chest strap should be placed in direct contact with the skin.

3. When properly placed, the digital display should provide HR values that update regularly (within seconds).

Sample Calculations

Gender: _Female_

Age: _24 years_

Resting heart rate count (radial pulse) for 30 seconds: _38 beats_

Step 1: Calculate the resting heart rate in beats per minute (bpm).

38 beats x 2 = 76 bpm

Step 2: Compare the resting heart rate (bpm) to the norms in table 2.1.

A score of 76 bpm would be classified as "> Average" for a woman, according to table 2.1.

REFERENCES

1. Adams, G. M. *Exercise Physiology: Laboratory Manual,* 4th edition. Boston: McGraw Hill, 2002.
2. Couldry, W. C., Corbin, C. B., and Wilcox, A. Carotid vs. radial pulse counts. *Phys. Sportsmed.* 10(12): 67–72, 1982.
3. Cramer, J. T., and Coburn, J. W. Fitness testing protocols and norms. In *NSCA's Essentials of Personal Training,* eds. R. W. Earle and T. R. Baechle. Champaign, IL: Human Kinetics, 2005, pp. 218–263.
4. Heyward, V. H. *Advanced Fitness Assessment and Exercise Prescription,* 4th edition. Champaign, IL: Human Kinetics, 2002.
5. McArdle, W. D., Katch, F. I., and Katch, V. L. *Exercise Physiology: Energy, Nutrition, and Human Performance,* 6th edition. Philadelphia: Lippincott Williams & Wilkins, 2007.
6. Oldridge, N. B., Haskell, W. L., and Single, P. Carotid palpation, coronary heart disease and exercise rehabilitation. *Med. Sci. Sports Exerc.* 13(1): 6–8, 1981.
7. Sedlock, D. A., Knowlton, R. G., Fitzgerald, P. I., Tahamont, M. V., and Schneider, D. A. Accuracy of subject-palpated carotid pulse after exercise. *Phys. Sportsmed.* 11(4): 106–116, 1983.
8. White, J. R. EKG changes using carotid artery for heart rate monitoring. *Med. Sci. Sports Exerc.* 9: 88, 1977.

RESTING HEART RATE FORM | Worksheet **2.1**

Name _____   Date _____

Gender: _____Male_____

Age: _____22_____

30-second radial pulse count: _____33_____

1. Resting heart rate (bpm)   = _____~~~~ 66_____

2. Resting heart rate classification = ~~~~~~ (see table 2.1)
   _____Average_____

EXTENSION ACTIVITIES | Worksheet **2.2**

Name _____   Date _____

Use the following data with table 2.1 to answer the questions below.

Gender: _____Female_____

Age: _____32 years_____

30-second radial pulse count: _____41 beats_____

1. Calculate the subject's resting heart rate.

   Resting heart rate (bpm)   = _____64_____

2. Classify the subject's resting heart rate based on table 2.1.

   Resting heart rate classification = _____Average_____

BACKGROUND

In addition to measuring heart rate, physical fitness assessments may involve the measurement of another basic vital sign: blood pressure (BP). Blood pressure is commonly defined as a measurement of the force of the blood acting against the vessel walls during and between heartbeats.[2] The pressure exerted against the vessels during a heartbeat (systole) is called the *systolic blood pressure,* while the pressure recorded between heartbeats (diastole) is called the *diastolic blood pressure.* The BP measurement is a combination of both the systolic and diastolic pressure and is usually written as "systolic / diastolic" (e.g., 120 / 80). BP is usually measured in units of millimeters of mercury (mm Hg). A common and normal BP measurement would be written as 120 / 80 mmHg.

Sounds are emitted as a result of the pressure exerted against the vessel walls, and these sounds are called Korotkoff sounds. The detection and disappearance of Korotkoff sounds when external pressure is applied provides the basis of traditional BP assessments. Sphygmomanometry is the most common and clinically acceptable technique to measure BP.[4] The American Heart Association regards the mercury sphygmomanometer (photo 3.1) as the gold standard measurement device for clinical BP assessment.[4] However, other techniques, such as aneroid (pressure gauge) and automated (photo 3.2) sphygmomanometers, are increasingly common, but these may be more prone to errors than mercury sphygmomanometers.[4] Nevertheless, with either mercury or aneroid sphygmomanometry, auscultation with a stethoscope placed

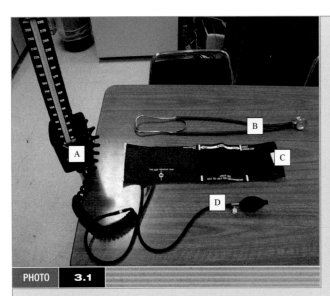

PHOTO **3.1**

A mercury sphygmomanometer. (A) Mercury column with pressure gradients listed from 0 to 300 mmHg, (B) stethoscope, (C) cuff, (D) air bulb and pressure release valve for inflating the cuff.

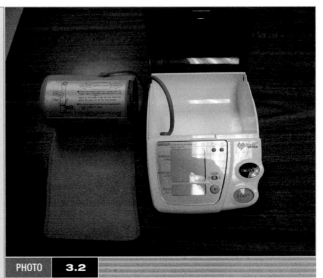

PHOTO **3.2**

An automated sphygmomanometer.

| | Classification of hypertension (JNC*-7). | TABLE | 3.1 |

Blood pressure classification	Systolic blood pressure (mmHg)	Diastolic blood pressure (mmHg)
Normal	< 120	< 80
Prehypertensive	120–139	80–89
Stage 1 hypertension	140–159	90–99
Stage 2 hypertension	≥ 160	≥ 100

Source: Pickering, T. G., Hall, J. E., Appel, L. J., Falkner, B. E., Graves, J., Hill, M. N., Jones, D. W., Kurtz, T., Sheps, S. G., and Roccella, E. J. Recommendations for blood pressure measurement in humans and experimental animals. Part 1: Blood pressure measurement in humans: A statement for professionals from the subcommittee of professional and public education of the American Heart Association Council on high blood pressure research. *Circulation* 111: 697–716, 2005, p. 700.

* Joint National Committee on Prevention, Detection, Evaluation, and Treatment of High Blood Pressure

over the brachial artery is necessary to hear the Korotkoff sounds. Therefore, sphygmomanometry is commonly called the "cuff," "auscultation," or "Korotkoff" technique.[4]

The premise of sphygmomanometry with auscultation is that the brachial artery is occluded with an air-inflated cuff placed around the arm (just distal to the shoulder). The amount of pressure used to inflate the cuff to occlude brachial artery blood flow should be greater than the individual's systolic BP.[4] As the cuff is deflated slowly, blood will eventually squeeze past the occlusion point (cuff) at a pressure that is equal to the systolic BP. A stethoscope is placed over the brachial artery distal to the cuff to auscultate the sounds made by the blood (i.e., Korotkoff sounds). The cuff pressure at which the first audible Korotkoff sounds occur while the cuff is deflating is denoted as the systolic BP, and the cuff pressure of the last audible Korotkoff sounds is recorded as the diastolic BP.

BP assessments are important for detecting hypertension (table 3.1) and monitoring the antihypertensive effects of an exercise program or dietary changes.[3] BP measurements are most often performed at rest (before exercise). BP can be assessed during and after exercise; however, these techniques require advanced skills for measurement and interpretation and will not be covered in this context.[1] The BP measurement technique described in this laboratory focuses on resting BP to evaluate the presence of hypertension and, consequently, the readiness of individuals to undergo other physical fitness tests. For example, if successive BP measurements indicate the possibility of hypertension (table 3.1) for an individual, then physical fitness testing may have to be postponed until medical clearance is granted by a physician. For more information on pre-exercise health status evaluations, see Lab 1.

KNOW THESE TERMS & ABBREVIATIONS

☐ auscultation = listening to sounds arising from organs to aid in diagnosis and treatment

☐ BP = blood pressure, measured in millimeters of mercury (mmHg). BP is defined as a measurement of the force of the blood acting against the vessel walls during and between heartbeats.

☐ systolic blood pressure = the pressure exerted against the vessels during a heartbeat (systole)

☐ diastolic blood pressure = the pressure recorded between heartbeats (diastole)

☐ Korotkoff sounds = the sounds emitted as a result of the pressure exerted against the vessel walls; these sounds provide the basis of traditional BP assessments

☐ sphygmomanometer = the instrument used to measure blood pressure in an artery, consisting of a pressure gauge and a rubber cuff, used with a stethoscope. Mercury and aneroid sphygmomanometers are available.

☐ hypertension = an abnormally high BP reading (≥ 140 / 90)

EQUIPMENT (see Appendix 2 for vendors)	**Approximate Price**
1. Mercury sphygmomanometer (photo 3.1)	$24–$40
2. Automated sphygmomanometer (photo 3.2)	$50–$100
3. Stethoscope (photo 3.1)	$21–$47
4. Tape measure (photo 3.3)	$7–$29

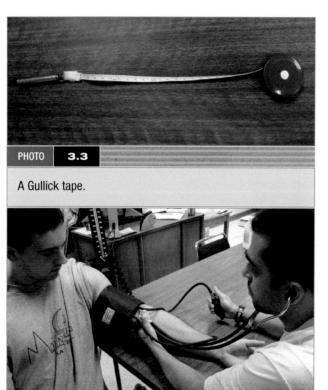

PHOTO **3.3**

A Gullick tape.

PHOTO **3.4**

Example of mercury sphygmomanometry with auscultation by the tester (right) controlling the air bulb for inflation/deflation of the cuff while monitoring the mercury column (upper left).

PROCEDURES

Mercury Sphygmomanometry (Auscultation Technique)[3,4]

1. To prepare for a resting BP assessment, the subject should be relaxed and comfortably seated upright with the legs uncrossed and the back and arms supported (photo 3.4). All clothing that covers the location of the cuff should be removed. The room temperature should be comfortable (not hot or cold), the environment should be free from distracting background noises, the subject's bladder should be relieved prior to the test, and no talking should be allowed by the subject or the tester during the test. Resting BP should always be taken prior to exercise, and caffeine, alcohol, and nicotine should be avoided for at least 30 minutes prior to any BP measurement.

2. Since various cuff sizes are available, the appropriate cuff size should be determined by measuring the arm circumference with a tape measure (photo 3.3) at 50% of the distance from the shoulder to the elbow. Once the arm circumference has been recorded, determine the appropriate BP cuff size with table 3.2.[4]

3. Place the cuff around the left or right arm so that the cuff is level with the heart. To do this, it is important to position the subject so that the arm is resting in the same horizontal plane

Determining cuff dimension using arm circumference.   **TABLE   3.2**

Size	Measured cuff dimensions	Measured arm circumference
Small adult	12 x 22 cm	22–26 cm
Adult	16 x 30 cm	27–34 cm
Large adult	16 x 36 cm	35–44 cm

as the heart. BP measurements taken with the arm hanging below or raised above the heart level will be inaccurate.[4] In addition, most cuffs have an identification line that is to be placed over the brachial artery. This feature allows the air bladder within the cuff to be positioned directly over the brachial artery. This is important for the occlusion of the artery during cuff inflation. Position the cuff so that the bottom edge of the cuff is approximately one inch (2.5 cm) above the antecubital space (elbow crease).

4. Once seated and relaxed, allow the subject to rest for at least five minutes prior to the first BP measurement.

5. With the subject's palm facing up, place the stethoscope head in the antecubital space firmly but not hard enough to indent the skin. It is recommended that the tester use his or her dominant hand to control the air bulb and the inflation/deflation of the cuff, while the nondominant hand should be used to hold the stethoscope (see photo 3.4; the tester is right-handed).

6. Assure that the mercury column (or aneroid pressure gauge) is easily readable by the tester. In photo 3.4, the mercury column is visible and at eye level for the tester. For aneroid pressure gauges, it is recommended to place the gauge in the tester's lap or clip it to the cuff to enable a quick and accurate pressure reading.

7. It is important to avoid contacting the stethoscope head with the air tubes connected to the mercury sphygmomanometer. If the air tubes contact the stethoscope head, the sound may be mistaken for a Korotkoff sound and may result in erroneous BP measurements. Therefore, position the air tubes away from the stethoscope head as much as possible.

8. Once the cuff, stethoscope, and sphygmomanometer have been properly placed, make sure the air release valve is closed on the air bulb and then quickly inflate the cuff either to 160 mmHg or to 20 mmHg above the anticipated systolic BP.

9. Upon reaching the maximum inflation pressure, carefully turn the air release valve counterclockwise to release the cuff pressure. The rate of pressure release should be approximately 2 to 3 mmHg per second.

10. While the cuff is deflating, listen carefully for the Korotkoff sounds. Record the systolic BP as an even number to the nearest 2 mmHg where the first Korotkoff sound is heard. Record the diastolic BP as an even number to the nearest 2 mmHg where the last Korotkoff sound is heard. Usually, Korotkoff sounds are described as sharp tapping noises

that are similar to tapping the stethoscope head (bell) gently with a finger. After the Korotkoff sounds have disappeared, observe the mercury column for another 10 to 20 mmHg of deflation to confirm the absence of sounds.

11. When it is confirmed that no more Korotkoff sounds are audible, rapidly deflate and remove the cuff.

12. After a minimum of two minutes of rest, measure BP again using the same technique described above. If the two consecutive measurements of either systolic BP or diastolic BP differ by more than 5 mmHg, take a third BP measurement. After either two or three consecutive BP measurements, calculate the average systolic and diastolic BP. The average systolic and diastolic BP values should be used as the final scores.

Automated Sphygmomanometry

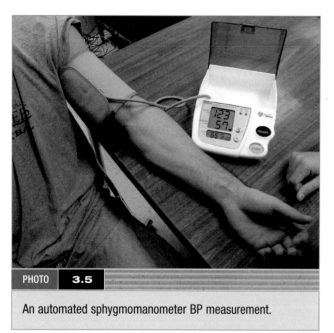

PHOTO   3.5

An automated sphygmomanometer BP measurement.

The American Heart Association recommends that any BP measurement technique other than mercury sphygmomanometry (including automated systems) should be validated prior to being used in practice.[4] Substantial errors in BP measurements and erroneous values may occur in both validated and unvalidated devices, but the probability of errors is reduced with validation.[4]

Most automated sphygmomanometers operate very similarly to the regular auscultation technique described above, except that a stethoscope is not required. Subject positioning and cuff placement are usually the same. Therefore, steps 1–4 and step 12 (above) may be applied. Because individual manufacturers may have different procedures, the manufacturer's directions should be carefully followed for any automated BP assessments. Photo 3.5 shows an automated sphygmomanometer BP assessment.

Sample Calculations

Gender: _Male_

Age: _19 years_

BLOOD PRESSURE	TRIAL 1	TRIAL 2	TRIAL 3
systolic (mmHg) =	124	118	118
diastolic (mmHg) =	72	66	70

Step 1: Calculate the average systolic and diastolic blood pressure values.

systolic: (124 + 118 + 118) ÷ 3 = 120

diastolic: (72 + 66 + 70) ÷ 3 = 69.3

final blood pressure = 120 / 69.3 mmHg

Step 2: Classify the final blood pressure measurement using table 3.1.

A score of 120 / 69.3 mmHg would be classified as normal in table 3.1.

BLOOD PRESSURE FORM   Worksheet **3.1**

Name   Mohamed Magano   Date 10-5 2023

Gender: Male

Age: 21

BLOOD PRESSURE:	TRIAL 1	TRIAL 2	TRIAL 3
Systolic (mmHg)	118	86	102
Diastolic (mmHg)	71	59	73

1. Final resting blood pressure (mmHg) = ~~109~~ 102/68

2. Resting blood pressure classification = Normal   (see table 3.1)

Pulse : 80

$$(118 + 86) \div 2 = \underline{106}$$

$$73+ 71 +59 \div 2 = 65$$

$$\frac{102}{68}$$

EXTENSION ACTIVITIES   Worksheet **3.2**

Name   Date

Use the following data with table 3.1 to answer the questions below.

Gender: Female

Age: 32 years

BLOOD PRESSURE:	TRIAL 1	TRIAL 2	TRIAL 3
Systolic (mmHg)	136	130	132
Diastolic (mmHg)	78	84	82

1. Calculate the subject's blood pressure.

   Final resting blood pressure (mmHg) = 109/71

2. Classify the subject's blood pressure based on table 3.1.

   Resting blood pressure classification = Normal   (see table 3.1)

REFERENCES

1. American College of Sports Medicine. *ACSM's Guidelines for Exercise Testing and Prescription,* 7th edition. Philadelphia: Lippincott Williams & Wilkins, 2006.

2. Adams, G. M. *Exercise Physiology: Laboratory Manual,* 4th edition. Boston: McGraw Hill, 2002.

3. Cramer, J. T., and Coburn, J. W. Fitness testing protocols and norms. In *NSCA's Essentials of Personal Training,* eds. R. W. Earle and T. R. Baechle. Champaign, IL: Human Kinetics, 2005, pp. 218–263.

4. Pickering, T. G., Hall, J. E., Appel, L. J., Falkner, B. E., Graves, J., Hill, M. N., Jones, D. W., Kurtz, T., Sheps, S. G., and Roccella, E. J. Recommendations for blood pressure measurement in humans and experimental animals. Part 1: Blood pressure measurement in humans: A statement for professionals from the subcommittee of professional and public education of the American Heart Association Council on high blood pressure research. *Circulation* 111: 697–716, 2005.

Unit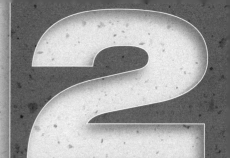

AEROBIC FITNESS

BACKGROUND

The determination of maximal oxygen consumption rate ($\dot{V}O_2$ max) provides information related to an individual's level of cardiorespiratory fitness and is a valuable predictor of endurance exercise and sports performance. In Lab 5, the Astrand–Rhyming submaximal cycle ergometer test utilizes the relationship between heart rate and power output to estimate $\dot{V}O_2$ max. In this laboratory, regression equations for males and females are used to estimate $\dot{V}O_2$ max without the need for subjects to exercise. The equations in this laboratory utilize demographic variables such as age, height, and body weight as well as descriptive variables related to exercise habits, including the duration of exercise, intensity of exercise, and years of training. Typically, the errors associated with these equations (± 10 to 15 percent) are approximately the same as those for exercise-based estimates of $\dot{V}O_2$ max.[1,2,3] The accuracy of the equations, however, is influenced by the level of fitness of the subject and, therefore, in this laboratory equations are provided that can be used for untrained as well as aerobically trained individuals.

KNOW THESE TERMS & ABBREVIATIONS

- ☐ R = multiple correlation coefficient; a numerical measure of how well a dependent variable can be predicted from a combination of independent variables (a number between −1 and 1)
- ☐ regression equations = statistical methods that are developed and used to relate two or more variables
- ☐ SEE = standard error of estimate; a measure of the accuracy of the predictions made using a regression equation
- ☐ $\dot{V}O_2$ max = maximal oxygen consumption rate

EQUIPMENT (see Appendix 2 for vendors)	Approximate Price
1. Meter stick	$10
2. Scale	$175
3. RPE scale	$18

PROCEDURES

Record the following information on Worksheet 4.1.

1. Your height in cm, body weight in kg, and age in years.
2. Refer to the Borg Rating of Perceived Exertion Scale (refer to figure 14.1 on p. 96) to estimate the typical intensity of training using the following statement:[2,3] "Indicate, in general, the intensity at which you perform your exercise regimen."

3. Indicate the duration of training using the following question:[2,3] "How many hours per week do you exercise?"

4. Record the years of training using the following question:[2,3] "How long have you consistently, no more than one month without exercise, been exercising?"

5. Determine the natural log of years of training.

6. Determine $\dot{V}O_2$ max in L • min⁻¹ or mL • min⁻¹

7. Calculate $\dot{V}O_2$ max in mL • kg⁻¹ • min⁻¹ using the relevant equation below.

8. Identify fitness category from table 4.1 on p. 25.

Equations

Untrained Males[1]

$\dot{V}O_2$ max (L • min⁻¹) = (0.046 (height in cm)) − (0.021 (age in years)) − 4.31

R (multiple correlation coefficient) = 0.87

SEE = 0.458 L • min⁻¹

Untrained Females[1]

$\dot{V}O_2$ max (L • min⁻¹) = (0.046 (height in cm)) − (0.021 (age in years)) − 4.93

R = 0.87

SEE = 0.458 L • min⁻¹

*Aerobically Trained Males[3]

$\dot{V}O_2$ max (mL • min⁻¹) = (27.387 (body weight in kg)) + (26.634 (height in cm)) − (27.572 (age in years)) + (26.161 (duration of training in hours per week)) + (114.904 (intensity of training using the Borg Scale)) + (506.752 (natural log of years of training)) − 4609.791

R = 0.82

SEE = 378 mL • min⁻¹

*Aerobically Trained Females[2]

$\dot{V}O_2$ max (mL • min⁻¹) = (18.528 (body weight in kg)) + (11.993 (height in cm)) − (17.197 (age in years)) + (23.522 (duration of training in hours per week)) + (62.118 (intensity of training using the Borg Scale)) + (278.262 (natural log of years of training)) − 1375.878

R = 0.83

SEE = 247 mL • min⁻¹

*Aerobically trained is defined as having participated in continuous aerobic exercise three or more sessions per week for a minimum of one hour per session, for at least the past 18 months.[2,3]

Sample Calculations

AEROBICALLY TRAINED MALE[3]

Height: _____180 cm_____

Body weight: _____80 kg_____

Age: _____25 years_____

Intensity of training: _____15_____

Duration of training: __6 h • wk^{-1}__

Years of training: __8 yr__ : natural log of 8 = 2.08

Equation: 27.387 × 80 = 2190.96

plus   26.634 × 180 = 6985.08

minus   27.572 × 25 = 6295.78

plus   26.161 × 6 = 6452.75

plus   114.904 × 15 = 8176.31

plus   506.752 × 2.08 = 9230.35

minus   4609.791 = $\dot{V}O_2$ max (mL • min^{-1}) = 4620.56 mL • min^{-1}

$\dot{V}O_2$ max (mL • kg^{-1} • min^{-1}) = 4620.56/80 = 57.76 mL • kg^{-1} • min^{-1}

Fitness category from table 4.1 = Superior

UNTRAINED FEMALE[1]

Height: ___166 cm___

Body weight: ___59 kg___

Age: __22 years__

Equation: 0.046 × 166 = 7.64

minus   0.021 × 22 = 7.18

minus   4.93 = $\dot{V}O_2$ max (L • min^{-1}) = 2.25 L • min^{-1}

$\dot{V}O_2$ max (mL • min^{-1}) = 2.25 × 1000 = 2250 mL • min^{-1}

$\dot{V}O_2$ max (mL • kg^{-1} • min^{-1}) = 2250 / 59 = 38.14 mL • kg^{-1} • min^{-1}

Fitness category from 4.1 = Excellent

Men's and women's aerobics fitness classification (predicted).[3]   **TABLE   4.1**

MEN		Age (years)					
Category	Measure	13–19	20–29	30–39	40–49	50–59	60+
I. Very Poor	$\dot{V}O_2$ max (mL • kg^{-1} • min^{-1})	<35.0	<33.0	<31.5	<30.2	<26.1	<20.5
II. Poor	$\dot{V}O_2$ max (mL • kg^{-1} • min^{-1})	35.0–38.3	33.0–36.4	31.5–35.4	30.2–33.5	26.1–30.9	20.5–26.0
III. Fair	$\dot{V}O_2$ max (mL • kg^{-1} • min^{-1})	38.4–45.1	36.5–42.4	35.5–40.9	33.6–38.9	31.0–35.7	26.1–32.2
IV. Good	$\dot{V}O_2$ max (mL • kg^{-1} • min^{-1})	45.2–50.9	42.5–46.4	41.0–44.9	39.0–43.7	35.8–40.9	32.2–36.4
V. Excellent	$\dot{V}O_2$ max (mL • kg^{-1} • min^{-1})	51.0–55.9	46.5–52.4	45.0–49.4	43.8–48.0	41.0–45.3	36.5–44.2
VI. Superior	$\dot{V}O_2$ max (mL • kg^{-1} • min^{-1})	>56.0	>52.5	>49.5	>48.1	>45.4	>44.3

WOMEN		Age (years)					
Category	Measure	13–19	20–29	30–39	40–49	50–59	60+
I. Very Poor	$\dot{V}O_2$ max (mL • kg^{-1} • min^{-1})	<25.0	<23.6	<22.8	<21.0	<20.2	<17.5
II. Poor	$\dot{V}O_2$ max (mL • kg^{-1} • min^{-1})	25.0–30.9	23.6–28.9	22.8–26.9	21.0–24.4	20.2–22.7	17.5–20.1
III. Fair	$\dot{V}O_2$ max (mL • kg^{-1} • min^{-1})	31.0–34.9	29.0–32.9	27.0–31.4	24.5–28.9	22.8–26.9	20.2–24.4
IV. Good	$\dot{V}O_2$ max (mL • kg^{-1} • min^{-1})	35.0–38.9	33.0–36.9	31.50–35.6	29.0–32.8	27.0–31.4	24.5–30.2
V. Excellent	$\dot{V}O_2$ max (mL • kg^{-1} • min^{-1})	39.0–41.9	37.0–40.9	35.7–40.0	32.9–36.9	31.5–35.7	30.3–31.4
VI. Superior	$\dot{V}O_2$ max (mL • kg^{-1} • min^{-1})	>42.0	>41.0	>40.1	>37.0	>35.8	>31.5

Source: Cooper, Kenneth H. *The Aerobics Way.* Toronto: Bantam Books, 1977, pp. 280–281. Printed with permission of Kenneth H. Cooper, MD, MPH, www.cooperaerobics.com.

Worksheet 4.1 — NON-EXERCISE-BASED ESTIMATION OF $\dot{V}O_2$ MAX

Name _____ Date _____

height = _17_ cm   intensity of training (from Borg scale) = _8_   years of training = _8_ yr
body weight = _66_ kg   duration of training = _2_ hr • wk^{-1} natural log of years of training = _____
age = _21_ yr

Equations

Untrained Male

0.046 × height = _____
minus   0.021 × age = _____
minus   4.31 = $\dot{V}O_2$ max (L • min^{-1}) = _____ L • min^{-1}
$\dot{V}O_2$ max (mL • min^{-1}) = _____ × 1000 = _____ mL • min^{-1}
$\dot{V}O_2$ max mL • kg^{-1} • min^{-1} = _____ / body weight = _____ mL • kg^{-1} • min^{-1}
Fitness category (table 4.1, page 25) = _____

Untrained Female

0.046 × height = _____
minus   0.021 × age = _____
minus   4.93 = $\dot{V}O_2$ max (L • min^{-1}) = _____ L • min^{-1}
$\dot{V}O_2$ max (mL • min^{-1}) = _____ × 1000 = _____ mL • min^{-1}
$\dot{V}O_2$ max (mL • kg^{-1} • min^{-1}) = _____ / body weight = _____ mL • kg^{-1} • min^{-1}
Fitness category (table 4.1) = _____

Aerobically Trained Male

27.387 × body weight = _66_
plus   26.634 × height = _172_
minus   27.572 × age = _21_
plus   26.161 × duration of training = _2_
plus   114.904 × intensity of training = _8_
plus   506.752 × natural log of years of training = _____
minus   4609.791 = $\dot{V}O_2$ max (mL • min^{-1}) = _____ mL • min^{-1}
$\dot{V}O_2$ max (mL • kg^{-1} • min^{-1}) = _623_ / body weight = _66_ mL • kg^{-1} • min^{-1}
Fitness category (table 4.1) = _44_

Aerobically Trained Female

18.528 × body weight = _____
plus   11.993 × height = _____
minus   17.197 × age = _____
plus   23.522 × duration of training = _____
plus   62.118 × intensity of training = _____
plus   278.262 × natural log of years of training = _____
minus   1375.878 = $\dot{V}O_2$ max (mL • min^{-1}) = _____ mL • min^{-1}
$\dot{V}O_2$ max (mL • kg^{-1} • min^{-1}) = _____ /body weight = _____ mL • kg^{-1} • min^{-1}
Fitness category (table 4.1) = _____

Name _____   *Date* _____

1. Given the following data: (a) calculate $\dot{V}O_2$ max in L • min⁻¹, mL • min⁻¹, and mL • kg⁻¹ • min⁻¹, and (b) determine the individual's fitness category from table 4.1 (page 25).

    untrained male

    height = 175 cm

    body weight = 78 kg

    age = 30 yr

    $\dot{V}O_2$ max (L • min⁻¹) = _____ L • min⁻¹

    $\dot{V}O_2$ max (mL • min⁻¹) = _____ mL • min⁻¹

    $\dot{V}O_2$ max (mL • kg⁻¹ • min⁻¹) = _____ mL • kg⁻¹ • min⁻¹

    Fitness category (table 4.1) = _____

2. Given the following data: (a) calculate $\dot{V}O_2$ max in mL • min⁻¹ and mL • kg⁻¹ • min⁻¹, and (b) determine the individual's fitness category from table 4.1.

    aerobically trained female

    height = 169 cm

    body weight = 65 kg

    age = 27 yr

    intensity of training = 14

    duration of training = 9 h • wk⁻¹

    years of training = 6 yr

    $\dot{V}O_2$ max (mL • min⁻¹) = _____ mL • min⁻¹

    $\dot{V}O_2$ max (mL • kg⁻¹ • min⁻¹) = _____ mL • kg⁻¹ • min⁻¹

    Fitness category (table 4.1) = _____

EXTENSION QUESTIONS

1. What are some common mistakes that may occur in administering this lab?

2. Identify possible sources of error in this lab.

3. Assess the practicality of using this lab in the field.

4. Research the reliability and/or validity of this lab using the Internet, journal articles, and other credible sources.

REFERENCES

1. Jones, N. L., Makrides, L., Hitchcock, C., Chypchar, T., and McCartney, N. Normal standards for an incremental progressive cycle ergometer test. *Am. Rev. Respir. Dis.* 131: 700–708, 1985.

2. Malek, M. H., Housh, T. J., Berger, D. E., Coburn, J. W., and Beck, T. W. A new non-exercise based $\dot{V}O_2max$

equation for aerobically trained females. *Med. Sci. Sports Exerc.* 36: 1804–1810, 2004.

3. Malek, M. H., Housh, T. J., Berger, D. E., Coburn, J. W., and Beck, T. W. A new non-exercise based $\dot{V}O_2max$ prediction equation for aerobically trained men. *J. Strength Cond. Res.* 19:559–565, 2005.

BACKGROUND

Endurance capabilities are reflected in one's ability to take in and utilize oxygen. Oxygen is a crucial factor in the operation of the electron transport system, where the production of large quantities of adenosine triphosphate (ATP) occurs as a result of oxidative metabolism. The ability to sustain moderate to high-intensity exercise for appreciable lengths of time is based on the rate at which ATP can be produced by oxidative means. Consequently, this rate will be reflected by the rate at which oxygen is consumed (taken in and utilized): oxygen consumption rate or $\dot{V}O_2$. One means of describing the cardiorespiratory endurance fitness level of an individual is by determining maximal oxygen consumption rate ($\dot{V}O_2$ max).

As one performs heavier power outputs on a cycle ergometer, both oxygen consumption rate and heart rate (HR) increase. Oxygen consumption rate increases because the demands of the work require increased production of energy and increased HR to transport oxygen and fuels to the active muscle tissues and remove their metabolic waste products more rapidly. The relationship of power output to oxygen consumption rate remains fairly constant between individuals, as well as within an individual at different times. Therefore, when we know the power output, the corresponding oxygen consumption rate can be predicted with reasonable accuracy ($\pm$ about 10 percent). However, the proportion to which HR increases in comparison to either power output or oxygen consumption rate will vary between individuals or within an individual based on level of fitness (endurance capability).

The ability to predict $\dot{V}O_2$ max is based on the fact that the heart pumps more efficiently and oxygen is more readily utilized for metabolism in individuals with higher maximal oxygen consumption capabilities. We can refer to this as increased cardiovascular efficiency, since the heart doesn't have to work as hard (HR is lower) to meet the metabolic demands of a task. Therefore, if two individuals are performing at the same power output (requiring the same rate of oxygen consumption), the individual with the higher $\dot{V}O_2$ max will tend to have a lower HR. The basis of the Astrand–Rhyming Test (named for the distinguished scientists who developed the test, P. O. Astrand and his wife, I. Rhyming) is to make use of this relationship.[2]

In essence, we would expect that if two individuals were to work such that similar HRs result (say 150 bpm), the individual with a higher $\dot{V}O_2$ max will actually be performing more physical work (again, this reflects cardiovascular efficiency). Therefore, the basic procedure of the test is to have an individual work at moderate intensity (HR = 120 – 170 bpm) and record both the HR and the power output. Using these two pieces of data, we can estimate $\dot{V}O_2$ max ($\pm$ 10 to 15 percent error) from previously determined relationships available in tables 5.1 and 5.2. This laboratory experience will help you become familiar with the procedures and supportive principles of this basic mode of fitness testing. In addition, you should be able to interpret the results of such testing in terms of fitness levels.

KNOW THESE TERMS & ABBREVIATIONS

☐ kgm • min^{-1} = kilogram meters per minute

☐ HR = heart rate

☐ $\dot{V}O_2$ = oxygen consumption rate; an indirect measure of aerobic energy production

☐ $\dot{V}O_2$ max = maximal oxygen consumption rate

EQUIPMENT (see Appendix 2 for vendors)	Approximate Price
1. Monark cycle ergometer	$2,000
2. Metronome	$175
3. Stopwatch	$10
4. HR monitor	$100

PROCEDURES

1. Set the seat height on the Monark cycle ergometer (see photo 5.1) for near full extension of the subject's legs while pedaling.

2. Have the subject warm up at 50 revolutions per minute (rpm) for three to five minutes at zero resistance. A metronome or digital pedal cadence recorder should be used to ensure proper rate of pedaling (see photo 5.2).

3. Set the first power output at 600 to 900 kgm • min^{-1} (approximately 100 to 150 watts). Determine this by multiplying the pedal cadence (always 50 for this test) • 6 (distance in meters the flywheel on the Monark cycle ergometer travels in one revolution) × resistance setting (see photo 5.3). Thus, a resistance setting of 2 kg at 50 rpm is equal to 600 kgm • min^{-1} (2 kg × 50 rpm × 6 m).

4. Start the six-minute test as soon as the correct pedaling cadence and power output are achieved (see photo 5.4).

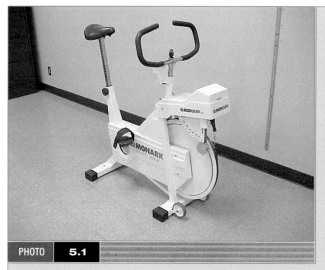

PHOTO **5.1**

Monark cycle ergometer.

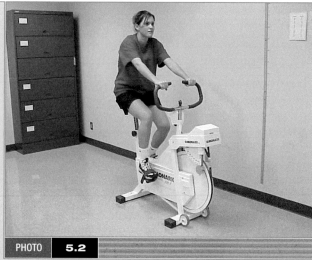

PHOTO **5.2**

Have the subject warm up at 50 rpm for three to five minutes at zero resistance.

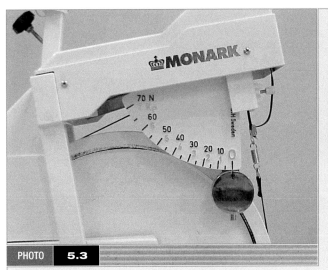

PHOTO **5.3**

Resistance setting on the Monark cycle ergometer.

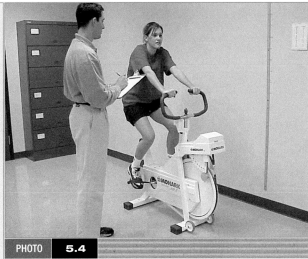

PHOTO **5.4**

Start the six-minute test as soon as the subject achieves the power output.

5. Measure and record the 30-second HR for the last 30 seconds of minutes 2 through 6.
6. At the end of the third minute, adjust the power output (up or down) if it is not likely that the subject will be in the target HR zone (120–170 bpm) at the end of the six-minute test.
7. If the subject has not reached a steady state HR by the end of the six minutes, extend the test until the difference between consecutive minutes is less than 10 bpm. The last two HR values should be averaged to use in calculations.
8. Allow the subject to cool down (see photo 5.5).

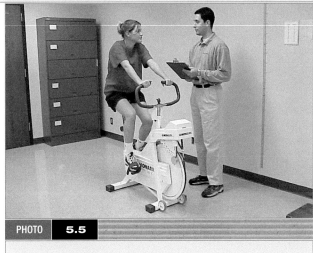

PHOTO **5.5**

Allow the subject to cool down.

Sample Calculations

If a 20-year-old, 154-pound male had an average HR of 150 bpm during the last two minutes of a 900 kgm • min^{-1} power output (3 kg resistance at 50 rpm), his values would be:

A. Preliminary $\dot{V}O_2$ max value from table 5.1 = 3.2 L • min^{-1}

B. 3.2 × 1.07 (age correction factor, table 5.3) = 3.425 L • min^{-1}

C. 3.425 L • min^{-1} × 1000 = 3425 mL • min^{-1}

D. $\dot{V}O_2$ max = (3425 mL • min^{-1}) / 70 kg = 48.9 mL • kg^{-1} • min^{-1}
(body weight = 154 lbs / 2.2046 = 70 kg)

E. Fitness category (table 5.4) = excellent

TABLE	5.1	Males' maximal oxygen consumption rate (L • min⁻¹) predicted from cycle ergometer test.[1]

	Power Output (kgm • min⁻¹)									
HR	150	300	450	600	750	900	1050	1200	1350	1500
120	1.6	2.2	2.8	3.5	4.1	4.8	5.6			
121	1.6	2.2	2.8	3.4	4.0	4.7	5.5			
122	1.6	2.2	2.8	3.4	4.0	4.6	5.4			
123		2.1	2.7	3.4	3.9	4.6	5.3			
124		2.1	2.7	3.3	3.9	4.5	5.2	6.0		
125		2.0	2.6	3.2	3.8	4.4	5.1	5.9		
126		2.0	2.6	3.2	3.8	4.4	5.1	5.8		
127		2.0	2.5	3.1	3.7	4.3	5.0	5.7		
128		2.0	2.5	3.1	3.6	4.2	4.9	5.6		
129		1.9	2.4	3.0	3.6	4.2	4.8	5.6		
130		1.9	2.4	3.0	3.5	4.1	4.8	5.5		
131		1.9	2.4	2.9	3.5	4.0	4.7	5.4		
132		1.8	2.3	2.9	3.4	4.0	4.6	5.3	6.0	
133		1.8	2.3	2.8	3.4	3.9	4.6	5.3	5.9	
134		1.8	2.3	2.8	3.3	3.9	4.5	5.2	5.8	
135		1.7	2.3	2.8	3.3	3.8	4.4	5.1	5.7	
136		1.7	2.2	2.7	3.2	3.8	4.4	5.0	5.6	
137		1.7	2.2	2.7	3.2	3.7	4.3	5.0	5.6	
138		1.6	2.2	2.7	3.2	3.7	4.3	4.9	5.5	
139		1.6	2.1	2.6	3.1	3.6	4.2	4.8	5.4	
140		1.6	2.1	2.6	3.1	3.6	4.2	4.8	5.4	6.0
141			2.1	2.6	3.0	3.5	4.1	4.7	5.3	5.9
142			2.1	2.5	3.0	3.5	4.1	4.6	5.2	5.8
143			2.0	2.5	2.9	3.4	4.0	4.6	5.2	5.7
144			2.0	2.5	2.9	3.4	4.0	4.5	5.1	5.7
145			2.0	2.4	2.9	3.4	3.9	4.5	5.0	5.6
146			2.0	2.4	2.8	3.3	3.9	4.4	5.0	5.6
147			2.0	2.4	2.8	3.3	3.8	4.4	4.9	5.5
148			1.9	2.4	2.8	3.2	3.8	4.3	4.9	5.4
149			1.9	2.3	2.7	3.2	3.7	4.3	4.8	5.4
150			1.9	2.3	2.7	3.2	3.7	4.2	4.8	5.3
151			1.9	2.3	2.7	3.1	3.7	4.2	4.7	5.2
152				2.3	2.7	3.1	3.6	4.1	4.6	5.2
153				2.2	2.6	3.0	3.6	4.1	4.6	5.1
154				2.2	2.6	3.0	3.5	4.0	4.5	5.1
155				2.2	2.6	3.0	3.5	4.0	4.5	5.0
156				2.2	2.5	2.9	3.4	4.0	4.4	5.0
157				2.1	2.5	2.9	3.4	3.9	4.4	4.9
158				2.1	2.5	2.9	3.4	3.9	4.3	4.9
159				2.1	2.4	2.8	3.3	3.8	4.3	4.8
160				2.1	2.4	2.8	3.3	3.8	4.3	4.8
161				2.0	2.4	2.8	3.2	3.7	4.2	4.7
162				2.0	2.4	2.8	3.2	3.7	4.2	4.6
163				2.0	2.4	2.8	3.2	3.7	4.2	4.6
164				2.0	2.3	2.7	3.1	3.6	4.1	4.5
165				2.0	2.3	2.7	3.1	3.6	4.1	4.5
166				1.9	2.3	2.7	3.1	3.6	4.1	4.5
167				1.9	2.2	2.6	3.0	3.5	4.0	4.4
168				1.9	2.2	2.6	3.0	3.5	4.0	4.4
169				1.9	2.2	2.6	3.0	3.5	3.9	4.3
170				1.8	2.2	2.6	3.0	3.4	3.9	4.3

Note: To convert kgm • min⁻¹ to watts, divide by 6.12.

From P.O. Astrand and K. Rodahl, *Textbook of Work Physiology.* Copyright © 1977 McGraw-Hill Book Company. Used with permission of the author.

Females' maximal oxygen consumption rate (L • min^{-1}) predicted from cycle ergometer test.[1]   TABLE   5.2

	Power Output (kgm • min^{-1})					
HR	150	300	450	600	750	900
120	1.8	2.6	3.4	4.1	4.8	
121	1.7	2.5	3.3	4.0	4.8	
122	1.7	2.5	3.2	3.9	4.7	
123	1.7	2.4	3.1	3.9	4.6	
124	1.7	2.4	3.1	3.8	4.5	
125	1.6	2.3	3.0	3.7	4.4	
126	1.6	2.3	3.0	3.6	4.3	
127	1.6	2.2	2.9	3.5	4.2	
128	1.6	2.2	2.8	3.5	4.2	4.8
129	1.6	2.2	2.8	3.4	4.1	4.8
130		2.1	2.7	3.4	4.0	4.7
131		2.1	2.7	3.4	4.0	4.6
132		2.0	2.7	3.3	3.9	4.5
133		2.0	2.6	3.2	3.8	4.4
134		2.0	2.6	3.2	3.8	4.4
135		2.0	2.6	3.1	3.7	4.3
136		1.9	2.5	3.1	3.6	4.2
137		1.9	2.5	3.0	3.6	4.2
138		1.8	2.4	3.0	3.5	4.1
139		1.8	2.4	2.9	3.5	4.0
140		1.8	2.4	2.8	3.4	4.0
141		1.8	2.3	2.8	3.4	3.9
142		1.7	2.3	2.8	3.3	3.9
143		1.7	2.2	2.7	3.3	3.8
144		1.7	2.2	2.7	3.2	3.8
145		1.6	2.2	2.7	3.2	3.7
146		1.6	2.2	2.6	3.2	3.7
147		1.6	2.1	2.6	3.1	3.6
148		1.6	2.1	2.6	3.1	3.6
149			2.1	2.6	3.0	3.5
150			2.0	2.5	3.0	3.5
151			2.0	2.5	3.0	3.4
152			2.0	2.5	2.9	3.4
153			2.0	2.4	2.9	3.3
154			2.0	2.4	2.8	3.3
155			1.9	2.4	2.8	3.2
156			1.9	2.3	2.8	3.2
157			1.9	2.3	2.7	3.2
158			1.8	2.3	2.7	3.1
159			1.8	2.2	2.7	3.1
160			1.8	2.2	2.6	3.0
161			1.8	2.2	2.6	3.0
162			1.8	2.2	2.6	3.0
163			1.7	2.2	2.6	2.9
164			1.7	2.1	2.5	2.9
165			1.7	2.1	2.5	2.9
166			1.7	2.1	2.5	2.8
167			1.6	2.1	2.4	2.8
168			1.6	2.0	2.4	2.8
169			1.6	2.0	2.4	2.8
170			1.6	2.0	2.4	2.7

Note: To convert kgm • min^{-1} to watts, divide by 6.12.

| TABLE | 5.3 | Age correction factors for predicting maximal oxygen consumption rate.[1] |

Age (yrs)	Correction Factor
20	1.07
25	1.00
35	0.87
45	0.78
55	0.71
65	0.65

From P.O. Astrand and K. Rodahl, *Textbook of Work Physiology.* Copyright © 1977 McGraw-Hill Book Company. Used with permission.

| TABLE | 5.4 | Men's and women's aerobics fitness classification (predicted).[3] |

MEN		Age (years)					
Category	Measure	13–19	20–29	30–39	40–49	50–59	60+
I. Very Poor	$\dot{V}O_2$ max (mL • kg^{-1} • min^{-1})	<35.0	<33.0	<31.5	<30.2	<26.1	<20.5
II. Poor	$\dot{V}O_2$ max (mL • kg^{-1} • min^{-1})	35.0–38.3	33.0–36.4	31.5–35.4	30.2–33.5	26.1–30.9	20.5–26.0
III. Fair	$\dot{V}O_2$ max (mL • kg^{-1} • min^{-1})	38.4–45.1	36.5–42.4	35.5–40.9	33.6–38.9	31.0–35.7	26.1–32.2
IV. Good	$\dot{V}O_2$ max (mL • kg^{-1} • min^{-1})	45.2–50.9	42.5–46.4	41.0–44.9	39.0–43.7	35.8–40.9	32.2–36.4
V. Excellent	$\dot{V}O_2$ max (mL • kg^{-1} • min^{-1})	51.0–55.9	46.5–52.4	45.0–49.4	43.8–48.0	41.0–45.3	36.5–44.2
VI. Superior	$\dot{V}O_2$ max (mL • kg^{-1} • min^{-1})	>56.0	>52.5	>49.5	>48.1	>45.4	>44.3

WOMEN		Age (years)					
Category	Measure	13–19	20–29	30–39	40–49	50–59	60+
I. Very Poor	$\dot{V}O_2$ max (mL • kg^{-1} • min^{-1})	<25.0	<23.6	<22.8	<21.0	<20.2	<17.5
II. Poor	$\dot{V}O_2$ max (mL • kg^{-1} • min^{-1})	25.0–30.9	23.6–28.9	22.8–26.9	21.0–24.4	20.2–22.7	17.5–20.1
III. Fair	$\dot{V}O_2$ max (mL • kg^{-1} • min^{-1})	31.0–34.9	29.0–32.9	27.0–31.4	24.5–28.9	22.8–26.9	20.2–24.4
IV. Good	$\dot{V}O_2$ max (mL • kg^{-1} • min^{-1})	35.0–38.9	33.0–36.9	31.50–35.6	29.0–32.8	27.0–31.4	24.5–30.2
V. Excellent	$\dot{V}O_2$ max (mL • kg^{-1} • min^{-1})	39.0–41.9	37.0–40.9	35.7–40.0	32.9–36.9	31.5–35.7	30.3–31.4
VI. Superior	$\dot{V}O_2$ max (mL • kg^{-1} • min^{-1})	>42.0	>41.0	>40.1	>37.0	>35.8	>31.5

Source: Cooper, Kenneth H. *The Aerobics Way.* Toronto: Bantam Books, 1977, pp. 280–281. Printed with permission of Kenneth H. Cooper, MD, MPH, www.cooperaerobics.com.

ASTRAND–RHYMING TEST FORM Worksheet **5.1**

Name _____   Date _____

Body weight _____   Gender _____

Minute	Heart rate for last 30 seconds of the time interval	Power output
1	_____	_____
2	_____	
3	_____	
4	_____	_____
5	_____	
6	_____	

Use if needed

7	_____	
8	_____	

Initial power output _____

Adjusted power output (if applicable) _____

Average HR for last two minutes of test _____

A. Preliminary $\dot{V}O_2$ max value from table 5.1 or 5.2 _____ $L \cdot min^{-1}$

B. Multiply preliminary $\dot{V}O_2$ max value by age correction factor (table 5.3) _____ $L \cdot min^{-1}$

C. Multiply $\dot{V}O_2$ max in $L \cdot min^{-1} \times 1000$ _____ $mL \cdot min^{-1}$

D. Divide the age-corrected $\dot{V}O_2$ max ($mL \cdot min^{-1}$) value by body weight in kg _____ $mL \cdot kg^{-1} \cdot min^{-1}$

E. Fitness category (table 5.4)[3] _____

Worksheet 5.2 | EXTENSION ACTIVITIES

Name _____   *Date* _____

1. A 20-year-old male (175 lbs) performed a submaximal cycle ergometer test. The following power outputs and heart rates were recorded. Using the blank graph below, predict this individual's maximal oxygen consumption rate ($\dot{V}O_2$ max). Assume a maximal HR of 200 bpm (220 − age = maximal HR) and express your answer relative to body weight (mL • kg^{-1} • min^{-1}). $\dot{V}O_2$ max = _____ mL • kg^{-1} • min^{-1}

Power Output 1   (300 kgm • min^{-1}),
HR = 100 bpm

Power Output 2   (900 kgm • min^{-1}),
HR = 150 bpm

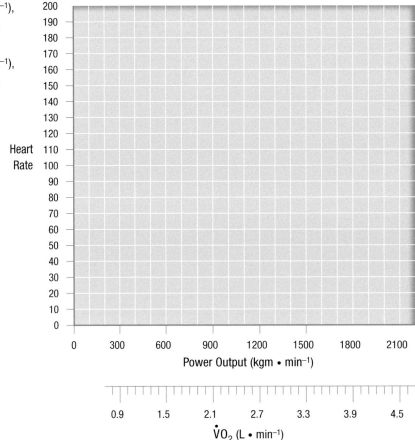

2. Activities such as weight training are not commonly used to estimate $\dot{V}O_2$ max. List at least one reason why this type of exercise would not accurately predict aerobic fitness.

3. Use your own data to calculate your estimated $\dot{V}O_2$ max (table 5.1 or 5.2) relative to your body weight (mL • kg^{-1} • min^{-1}) and determine your level of endurance fitness based on the classification from table 5.4.

EXTENSION QUESTIONS

1. What are some common mistakes that may occur in administering this lab?

2. Identify possible sources of error in this lab.

3. Assess the practicality of using this lab in the field.

4. Research the reliability and/or validity of this lab using the Internet, journal articles, and other credible sources.

REFERENCES

1. Astrand, P. O., and Rodahl, K. *Textbook of Work Physiology.* New York: McGraw-Hill Book Company, 1977, pp. 350–352.

2. Astrand, P. O., and Rhyming, I. A nomogram for calculation of aerobic capacity (physical fitness) from pulse rate during submaximal work. *J. Appl. Physiol.* 7: 218–221, 1954.

3. Cooper, K. H. *The Aerobics Way.* Toronto: Bantam Books, 1977, pp. 280–281.

BACKGROUND

The Queens College Step Test was designed to provide quick, easy, and accurate predictions of $\dot{V}O_2$ max for college-age men[1] and women.[1,2] This test involves only three minutes of stair stepping. Upon completion of the Queens College Step Test, the subject's heart rate is recorded, and this measurement is referred to as the recovery heart rate. In theory, individuals' recovery heart rate will be lower after the Queens College Step Test if they are in better shape (i.e., higher $\dot{V}O_2$ max), and individuals who exhibit poor fitness levels (i.e., lower $\dot{V}O_2$ max) will have a higher recovery heart rate after the step test. A higher recovery heart rate usually reflects a greater amount of exercise-induced stress as a result of the same submaximal stair-stepping task for all participants. Overall, the lower the post-exercise recovery heart rate, the higher the predicted $\dot{V}O_2$ max.

Perhaps the greatest advantages of the Queens College Step Test over other field-based cardiovascular tests (e.g., 12-minute run, 1.5-mile run, or Rockport fitness walking test) are: (a) it requires only three minutes of submaximal stair stepping and (b) large groups of individuals can be tested in a relatively short time. A common use of the test is to have a group of students organize into pairs. Half of the group performs the Queens College Step Test on a long bench, while the partner monitors and records the recovery heart rate. Upon completion of the first group, the pairs switch tasks so that all students are tested with only two three-minute step test sessions.

Here are the $\dot{V}O_2$ max prediction equations for the Queens College Step Test:

COLLEGE-AGE MEN[1]

$\dot{V}O_2$ max (mL • kg^{-1} • min^{-1}) = 111.33 – (0.42 × recovery heart rate in beats per minute)

COLLEGE-AGE WOMEN

$\dot{V}O_2$ max (mL • kg^{-1} • min^{-1}) = 65.81 – (0.1847 × recovery heart rate in beats per minute)

r (correlation coefficient) = –0.75

standardized error of prediction = 2.9 (mL • kg^{-1} • min^{-1})

KNOW THESE TERMS & ABBREVIATIONS

☐ recovery heart rate = the HR taken after the end of exercise (in this lab it is taken five seconds after the completion of the Queens College Step Test)

☐ regression equations = statistical methods that are developed and used to relate two or more variables

☐ $\dot{V}O_2$ max = maximal oxygen consumption rate

EQUIPMENT (see Appendix 2 for vendors) **Approximate Price**

1. Bench, stair step, or bleacher step that is 16.25″ (41.3 cm) tall $115
2. Metronome $20–$100
3. Stopwatch $10
4. Heart rate monitor $100

PROCEDURES[1,2] (see photos 6.1–6.5)

1. Have the subject (or group of subjects) warm up by walking briskly or jogging for five minutes prior to the test.
2. Instruct the subject (or group of subjects) to perform three minutes of stepping using a four-step cadence: "up–up–down–down." Ensure that the subjects are stepping with their entire feet on the bench/step and that the contralateral foot makes complete contact with the bench/step at the top (see photos 6.1–6.4). Encourage the participants to alternate legs, such that the consecutive stepping cycles would be performed as: right leg up, left leg up, right leg down, left leg down → right leg up, left leg up, right leg down, left leg down → right leg up, and so forth." Each step should be taken with each tick of the metronome, using the following cadences:
   a. Men will maintain a cadence of 24 steps per minute, which is equivalent to 96 beats per minute on a metronome.
   b. Women will complete 22 steps per minute, which is 88 beats per minute on a metronome.

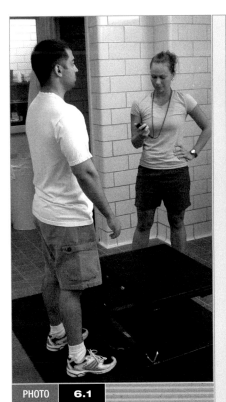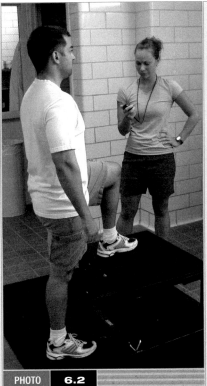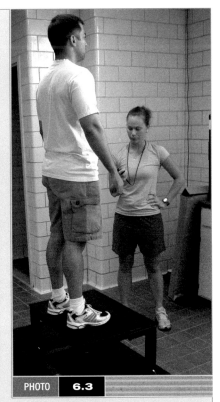

Ensure that subject steps with his entire feet on the step. One step should be taken with each tick of the metronome.

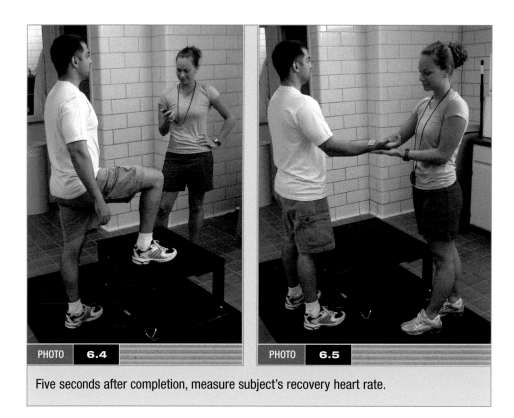

PHOTO 6.4 PHOTO 6.5

Five seconds after completion, measure subject's recovery heart rate.

3. Five seconds after the three-minute Queens College Step Test is complete, measure the subject's recovery heart rate (see photo 6.5) and record it (in beats per minute) on worksheet 6.1.

4. Use one of the regression equations below to predict $\dot{V}O_2$ max.

5. Compare the estimated $\dot{V}O_2$ max score to the norms listed in table 6.1.

Equations

COLLEGE-AGE MEN[1]

$\dot{V}O_2$ max (mL • kg^{-1} • min^{-1}) = 111.33 − (0.42 × recovery heart rate in beats per minute)

COLLEGE-AGE WOMEN

$\dot{V}O_2$ max (mL • kg^{-1} • min^{-1}) = 65.81 − (0.1847 × recovery heart rate in beats per minute)

Sample Calculations

Gender: _____Male_____

age: _19 years_

body weight: ___182 lbs___

recovery heart rate: ___150 bpm___

Step 1: Calculate the predicted $\dot{V}O_2$max.

$\dot{V}O_2$ max (mL • kg^{-1} • min^{-1}) = 111.33 − (0.42 × 150 bpm)

= 48.3 mL • kg^{-1} • min^{-1}

Step 2: Compare the predicted $\dot{V}O_2$ max score from the Queens College Step Test to the norms in table 6.1.

A score of 48.3 (mL • kg^{-1} • min^{-1}) would be classified as "good" for a 13- to 19-year-old man, according to table 6.1.

Men's and women's aerobic fitness classification (predicted).   **TABLE   6.1**

MEN		Age (years)					
Category	Measure	13–19	20–29	30–39	40–49	50–59	60+
I. Very Poor	$\dot{V}O_2$ max (mL • kg^{-1} • min^{-1})	<35.0	<33.0	<31.5	<30.2	<26.1	<20.5
II. Poor	$\dot{V}O_2$ max (mL • kg^{-1} • min^{-1})	35.0–38.3	33.0–36.4	31.5–35.4	30.2–33.5	26.1–30.9	20.5–26.0
III. Fair	$\dot{V}O_2$ max (mL • kg^{-1} • min^{-1})	38.4–45.1	36.5–42.4	35.5–40.9	33.6–38.9	31.0–35.7	26.1–32.2
IV. Good	$\dot{V}O_2$ max (mL • kg^{-1} • min^{-1})	45.2–50.9	42.5–46.4	41.0–44.9	39.0–43.7	35.8–40.9	32.2–36.4
V. Excellent	$\dot{V}O_2$ max (mL • kg^{-1} • min^{-1})	51.0–55.9	46.5–52.4	45.0–49.4	43.8–48.0	41.0–45.3	36.5–44.2
VI. Superior	$\dot{V}O_2$ max (mL • kg^{-1} • min^{-1})	>56.0	>52.5	>49.5	>48.1	>45.4	>44.3

WOMEN		Age (years)					
Category	Measure	13–19	20–29	30–39	40–49	50–59	60+
I. Very Poor	$\dot{V}O_2$ max (mL • kg^{-1} • min^{-1})	<25.0	<23.6	<22.8	<21.0	<20.2	<17.5
II. Poor	$\dot{V}O_2$ max (mL • kg^{-1} • min^{-1})	25.0–30.9	23.6–28.9	22.8–26.9	21.0–24.4	20.2–22.7	17.5–20.1
III. Fair	$\dot{V}O_2$ max (mL • kg^{-1} • min^{-1})	31.0–34.9	29.0–32.9	27.0–31.4	24.5–28.9	22.8–26.9	20.2–24.4
IV. Good	$\dot{V}O_2$ max (mL • kg^{-1} • min^{-1})	35.0–38.9	33.0–36.9	31.50–35.6	29.0–32.8	27.0–31.4	24.5–30.2
V. Excellent	$\dot{V}O_2$ max (mL • kg^{-1} • min^{-1})	39.0–41.9	37.0–40.9	35.7–40.0	32.9–36.9	31.5–35.7	30.3–31.4
VI. Superior	$\dot{V}O_2$ max (mL • kg^{-1} • min^{-1})	>42.0	>41.0	>40.1	>37.0	>35.8	>31.5

Source: Cooper, Kenneth H. *The Aerobics Way.* Toronto: Bantam Books, 1977, pp. 280–281. Printed with permission of Kenneth H. Cooper, MD, MPH, www.cooperaerobics.com.

Worksheet **6.1** QUEENS COLLEGE STEP TEST FORM

Name _____ Date _____

Gender: _____Male_____

Recovery heart rate (bpm): _____~~cross out~~ 110_____

1. Predicted $\dot{V}O_2$ max (mL • kg⁻¹ • min⁻¹) = _____44_____

2. Classification = _____Good_____ (see table 6.1)

X YMCA test

Worksheet **6.2** EXTENSION ACTIVITIES

Name _____ Date _____

Use the following data and table 6.1 to answer the questions below.

Gender: _____Female_____

Age: _____32 years_____

Recovery heart rate: _____187 bpm_____

1. Calculate the subject's predicted $\dot{V}O_2$max from the Queens College Step Test.
   $\dot{V}O_2$ max = _____ (mL • kg⁻¹ • min⁻¹)

2. Classify the subject's predicted $\dot{V}O_2$max from the Queens College Step Test (see table 6.1).
   Classification = _____

3. On the graph below, draw the expected relationship between recovery heart rate from the Queens College Step Test and $\dot{V}O_2$ max.

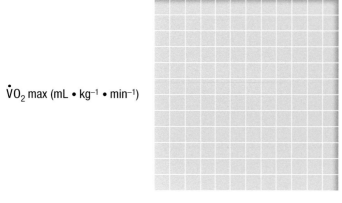

$\dot{V}O_2$ max (mL • kg⁻¹ • min⁻¹)

recovery heart rate

EXTENSION QUESTIONS

1. What are some common mistakes that may occur in administering this lab?

2. Identify possible sources of error in this lab.

3. Assess the practicality of using this lab in the field.

4. Research the reliability and/or validity of this lab using the Internet, journal articles, and other credible sources.

REFERENCES

1. McArdle, W. D., Katch, F. I., and Katch, V. L. *Exercise Physiology: Energy, Nutrition, and Human Performance,* 6th edition. Philadelphia: Lippincott Williams & Wilkins, 2007.

2. McArdle, W. D., Katch, F. I., Pechar, G. S., Jacobson, L., and Ruck, S. Reliability and interrelationships between maximal oxygen intake, physical work capacity and step-test scores in college women. *Med. Sci. Sports.* 4: 182–186, 1972.

Lab 7

Rockport Fitness Walking Test

BACKGROUND

The Rockport Fitness Walking Test (RFWT) was developed by Kline et al.[5] as a submaximal field test for predicting maximal oxygen consumption rate ($\dot{V}O_2$ max) using a one-mile walking protocol. During the RFWT, participants are instructed to walk for one mile as fast as possible while maintaining a constant pace. Immediately after the RFWT, heart rate (beats per minute) is assessed, and the time (minutes) to complete the one-mile walk is recorded. These variables, as well as body weight (lbs) and age (years), are then used in a regression equation to predict $\dot{V}O_2$ max. In theory, a lower post-exercise heart rate and time to complete the one-mile walk will result in a higher predicted $\dot{V}O_2$ max. Therefore, since the RFWT does not involve running or jogging, as in the 12-minute or 1.5-mile run tests, the RFWT may be appropriate for individuals with lower fitness levels or older adults who may not be able to run.

The original RFWT equations by Kline et al.[5] provided acceptable $\dot{V}O_2$ max predictions for men and women between the ages of 30 and 69 years. Fenstermaker et al.[3] cross-validated the RFWT equations for 65- to 79-year-old women and determined that the RFWT was appropriate for this population as well. However, other studies[2,4] have demonstrated that the original RFWT[5] consistently overpredicted $\dot{V}O_2$ max for college-aged men and women. Therefore, Dolgener et al.[2] modified the original RFWT equations to better predict $\dot{V}O_2$ max for 18- to 29-year-old men and women, and these modified equations have been validated by George et al.[4]

Since the applicable age range is broad (30–79 years) for the original equations by Kline et al.,[5] age is included as a predictor variable. However, the modified equations by Dolgener et al.[2] do not include age as a predictor, because the age range for these equations is narrow (18–29 years).

MEN (30–69 YEARS)[5]

$\dot{V}O_2$ max (mL • kg^{-1} • min^{-1}) = 139.168 – (0.3877 × age in years)
– (0.1692 × body weight in lbs) – (3.2649 × 1.0-mile walk time in min)
– (0.1565 × heart rate in beats per min)

R (multiple correlation coefficient) = 0.83–0.88

SEE (standard error of estimate) = 4.5–5.3 mL • kg^{-1} • min^{-1}

WOMEN (30–79 YEARS)[3,5]

$\dot{V}O_2$ max (mL • kg^{-1} • min^{-1}) = 132.853 – (0.3877 × age in years)
– (0.1692 × body weight in lbs) – (3.2649 × 1.0-mile walk time in min)
– (0.1565 × heart rate in beats per min)

R (multiple correlation coefficient) = 0.59–0.88

SEE (standard error of estimate) = 2.7–5.3 mL • kg^{-1} • min^{-1}

MEN (18–29 YEARS)[2,4]

$\dot{V}O_2$ max (mL • kg^{-1} • min^{-1}) = 97.660 – (0.0957 × body weight in lbs)
– (1.4537 × 1.0-mile walk time in min) – (0.1194 × heart rate in beats per min)

R (multiple correlation coefficient) = 0.50–0.85

SEE (standard error of estimate) = 3.5–5.8 mL • kg⁻¹ • min⁻¹

WOMEN (18–29 YEARS)[2,4]

$\dot{V}O_2$ max (mL • kg⁻¹ • min⁻¹) = 88.768 – (0.0957 × body weight in lbs)
– (1.4537 × 1.0-mile walk time in min) – (0.1194 × heart rate in beats per min)

R (multiple correlation coefficient) = 0.38–0.85

SEE (standard error of estimate) = 3.0–4.8 mL • kg⁻¹ • min⁻¹

KNOW THESE TERMS & ABBREVIATIONS

☐ RFWT = Rockport Fitness Walking Test

☐ R = multiple correlation coefficient: a numerical measure of how well a dependent variable can be predicted from a combination of independent variables (a number between –1 and 1)

☐ regression equations = statistical methods that are developed and used to relate two or more variables

☐ SEE = standard error of estimate: a measure of the accuracy of the predictions made using a regression equation

☐ $\dot{V}O_2$ max = maximal oxygen consumption rate

☐ 1 mile = 1.6 km

EQUIPMENT (see Appendix 2 for vendors)   Approximate Price

1. Measured 1.0-mile (1.6 kilometers) walking course that is flat and uninterrupted (e.g., 400-meter track)
2. Scale $175
3. Stopwatch $10
4. Heart rate monitor $100

PROCEDURES[1]

1. Measure body weight (in lbs) on a scale.
2. Have the subject (or group of subjects) warm up by walking briskly for five minutes prior to the test and put on the heart rate monitor (see photo 7.1).
3. Instruct the subject (or group of subjects) to walk briskly (i.e., as fast as possible) for 1.0 mile (1.6 km) while maintaining a constant pace (see photo 7.2).
4. Immediately after the 1.0-mile walk is complete, measure the subject's heart rate and record it (in beats per minute) on worksheet 7.1.
5. Measure the time it takes to complete the 1.0-mile walk and record it (in minutes) on worksheet 7.1.
6. Use one of the following regression equations to predict $\dot{V}O_2$ max.
7. Compare the estimated $\dot{V}O_2$ max score to the norms listed in table 7.1.

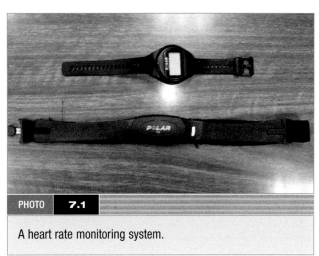

PHOTO **7.1**

A heart rate monitoring system.

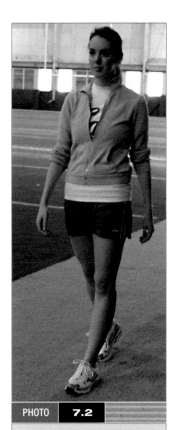

PHOTO **7.2**

Subject walking on the track to complete the Rockport Fitness Walking Test.

Equations

MEN (30–65 YEARS)

$\dot{V}O_2$ max (mL • kg^{-1} • min^{-1}) = 139.168 – (0.3877 × age in years) – (0.1692 × body weight in lbs) – (3.2649 × 1.0-mile walk time in min) – (0.1565 × heart rate in beats per min)

WOMEN (30–79 YEARS)

$\dot{V}O_2$ max (mL • kg^{-1} • min^{-1}) = 132.853 – (0.3877 × age in years) – (0.1692 × body weight in lbs) – (3.2649 × 1.0-mile walk time in min) – (0.1565 × heart rate in beats per min)

MEN (18–29 YEARS)

$\dot{V}O_2$ max (mL • kg^{-1} • min^{-1}) = 97.660 – (0.0957 × body weight in lbs) – (1.4537 × 1.0-mile walk time in min) – (0.1194 × heart rate in beats per min)

WOMEN (18–29 YEARS)

$\dot{V}O_2$ max (mL • kg^{-1} • min^{-1}) = 88.768 – (0.0957 × body weight in lbs) – (1.4537 × 1.0-mile walk time in min) – (0.1194 × heart rate in beats per min)

Sample Calculations

Gender: ___Female___

Age: __35 years__

Body weight: __138 lbs__

Post-walking heart rate: __118 bpm__

1.0-mile walk time: __15:54 min:sec__

Step 1: Convert time to minutes.

   54 sec / 60 sec = 0.9 min

Therefore,

   15:54 min:sec = 15.9 min

Step 2: Calculate the predicted $\dot{V}O_2$ max.

   $\dot{V}O_2$ max (mL • kg^{-1} • min^{-1})
   = 132.853 – (0.3877 × 35 years)
   – (0.1692 × 138 lbs) – (3.2649
   × 15.9 min) – (0.1565 × 118 bpm)
   = 25.6 mL • kg^{-1} • min^{-1}

Step 3: Compare the predicted $\dot{V}O_2$ max score from the Rockport Fitness Walking Test to the norms in table 7.1.

   A score of 25.6 mL • kg^{-1} • min^{-1} would be classified as "poor" for a 30- to 39-year-old woman in table 7.1.

Men's and women's aerobic fitness classification (predicted).   **TABLE** **7.1**

MEN		Age (years)					
Category	Measure	13–19	20–29	30–39	40–49	50–59	60+
I. Very Poor	$\dot{V}O_2$ max (mL • kg^{-1} • min^{-1})	<35.0	<33.0	<31.5	<30.2	<26.1	<20.5
II. Poor	$\dot{V}O_2$ max (mL • kg^{-1} • min^{-1})	35.0–38.3	33.0–36.4	31.5–35.4	30.2–33.5	26.1–30.9	20.5–26.0
III. Fair	$\dot{V}O_2$ max (mL • kg^{-1} • min^{-1})	38.4–45.1	36.5–42.4	35.5–40.9	33.6–38.9	31.0–35.7	26.1–32.2
IV. Good	$\dot{V}O_2$ max (mL • kg^{-1} • min^{-1})	45.2–50.9	42.5–46.4	41.0–44.9	39.0–43.7	35.8–40.9	32.2–36.4
V. Excellent	$\dot{V}O_2$ max (mL • kg^{-1} • min^{-1})	51.0–55.9	46.5–52.4	45.0–49.4	43.8–48.0	41.0–45.3	36.5–44.2
VI. Superior	$\dot{V}O_2$ max (mL • kg^{-1} • min^{-1})	>56.0	>52.5	>49.5	>48.1	>45.4	>44.3

WOMEN		Age (years)					
Category	Measure	13–19	20–29	30–39	40–49	50–59	60+
I. Very Poor	$\dot{V}O_2$ max (mL • kg^{-1} • min^{-1})	<25.0	<23.6	<22.8	<21.0	<20.2	<17.5
II. Poor	$\dot{V}O_2$ max (mL • kg^{-1} • min^{-1})	25.0–30.9	23.6–28.9	22.8–26.9	21.0–24.4	20.2–22.7	17.5–20.1
III. Fair	$\dot{V}O_2$ max (mL • kg^{-1} • min^{-1})	31.0–34.9	29.0–32.9	27.0–31.4	24.5–28.9	22.8–26.9	20.2–24.4
IV. Good	$\dot{V}O_2$ max (mL • kg^{-1} • min^{-1})	35.0–38.9	33.0–36.9	31.50–35.6	29.0–32.8	27.0–31.4	24.5–30.2
V. Excellent	$\dot{V}O_2$ max (mL • kg^{-1} • min^{-1})	39.0–41.9	37.0–40.9	35.7–40.0	32.9–36.9	31.5–35.7	30.3–31.4
VI. Superior	$\dot{V}O_2$ max (mL • kg^{-1} • min^{-1})	>42.0	>41.0	>40.1	>37.0	>35.8	>31.5

Source: Cooper, Kenneth H. *The Aerobics Way.* Toronto: Bantam Books, 1977, pp. 280–281. Printed with permission of Kenneth H. Cooper, MD, MPH, www.cooperaerobics.com.

Worksheet 7.1	ROCKPORT FITNESS WALKING TEST FORM

Name _____   *Date* _____

Gender: _____

Age (years): _____

Body weight (lbs): _____

Post-walking heart rate (bpm): _____

Time to complete the 1.0-mile walk (min:sec): _____

1. Time (in min:sec) to complete the 1.0-mile walk = _____ minutes

2. Predicted $\dot{V}O_2$ max (mL $\cdot$ kg^{-1} $\cdot$ min^{-1}) = _____

3. Classification = _____ (see table 7.1)

Worksheet 7.2	EXTENSION ACTIVITIES

Name _____   *Date* _____

Use the following data and table 7.1 to answer the questions below.

Gender: Male

Age: 19 years

Body weight: 185 lbs

Post-walking heart rate: 130 bpm

1.0-mile walk time: 14:46 min:sec

1. Calculate the subject's predicted $\dot{V}O_2$ max from the Rockport Fitness Walking Test.

   $\dot{V}O_2$ max = _____ (mL $\cdot$ kg^{-1} $\cdot$ min^{-1})

2. Classify the subject's predicted $\dot{V}O_2$ max from the Rockport Fitness Walking Test (see table 7.1).

   Classification = _____

EXTENSION QUESTIONS

1. What are some common mistakes that may occur in administering this lab?
2. Identify possible sources of error in this lab.
3. Assess the practicality of using this lab in the field.
4. Research the reliability and/or validity of this lab using the Internet, journal articles, and other credible sources.

REFERENCES

1. Cramer, J. T., and Coburn, J. W. Fitness testing protocols and norms. In *NSCA's Essentials of Personal Training*, eds. R. W. Earle and T. R. Baechle. Champaign, IL: Human Kinetics, 2005, pp. 218–263.

2. Dolgener, F. A., Hensley, L. D., Marsh, J. J., and Fjelstul, J. K. Validation of the Rockport fitness walking test in college males and females. *Res. Q. Exerc. Sport.* 65: 152–158, 1994.

3. Fenstermaker, K. L., Plowman, S. A., and Looney, M. A. Validation of the Rockport fitness walking test in females 65 years and older. *Res. Q. Exerc. Sport.* 63: 322–327, 1992.

4. George, J. D., Fellingham, G. W., and Fisher, A. G. A modified version of the Rockport fitness walking test for college men and women. *Res. Q. Exerc. Sport.* 69: 205–209, 1998.

5. Kline, G. M., Porcari, J. P., Hintermeister, R., Freedson, P. S., Ward, A., McCarron, R. F., Ross, J., and Rippe, J. M. Estimation of VO$_2$max from a one-mile track walk, gender, age and body weight. *Med. Sci. Sports Exerc.* 19: 253–259, 1987.

12-Minute Run Test

BACKGROUND

The 12-minute run test is a field test designed to predict maximal oxygen consumption rate ($\dot{V}O_2$ max) by measuring the distance completed in 12 minutes of running (or walking). Although walking is allowed during this test, the objective is to cover as much distance as possible in 12 minutes. A faster pace (speed) during the test will result in a greater distance covered, and, therefore, a higher predicted $\dot{V}O_2$ max. After the test is complete and the distance is recorded, it is used in the following regression equation[2] to predict $\dot{V}O_2$ max:

$\dot{V}O_2$ max (mL • kg^{-1} • min^{-1}) = [0.0268 • distance in meters completed in 12 minutes] – 11.3

r (correlation coefficient) = 0.897

The 12-minute run test was originally established based on an early study by Balke,[1] which led to the development of the regression equation used in this laboratory to predict $\dot{V}O_2$ max.[2] Based on the linear relationship between running velocity (from 150 to 300 m • min^{-1}) and steady-state $\dot{V}O_2$, Balke[1] found that a 12-minute "best effort" run closely estimated the $\dot{V}O_2$ max from a constant speed, graded walk test. When Cooper[2] developed the regression equation to predict $\dot{V}O_2$ max using the 12-minute run, a correlation coefficient of r = 0.897 was reported. Since then, Safrit et al.[8] have reported validity coefficients ranging from r = 0.28 to 0.94 for measured $\dot{V}O_2$ max versus predicted $\dot{V}O_2$ max from the 12-minute run test. It was later suggested, however, that the variation among these correlations may have been due to the type of criterion $\dot{V}O_2$ max test performed.[7] Nevertheless, most studies have agreed that $\dot{V}O_2$ max can be accurately predicted with the 12-minute run test.[2,4,6,7,8,9]

KNOW THESE TERMS & ABBREVIATIONS

- ☐ $\dot{V}O_2$ max = maximal oxygen consumption rate
- ☐ regression equations = statistical methods that are developed and used to relate two or more variables
- ☐ correlation coefficient (r) = a numerical measure of the degree to which two variables are linearly related (a number between –1 and 1)

EQUIPMENT (See Appendix 2 for vendors)   Approximate Price

1. A 400-meter track or premeasured flat course is recommended so that the distance covered in 12 minutes can be accurately determined.

2. Cones or markers to divide the course into quarters or eighths to accurately determine the distance completed during the 12-minute run test $10

3. Stopwatch $10

PROCEDURES[3]

1. Have the subject(s) warm up by walking and/or jogging for five minutes prior to the test.

2. Instruct the subject to run (or walk if necessary) as far as possible in 12 minutes. Emphasize that a faster speed will result in a higher predicted $\dot{V}O_2$ max.

3. Measure the distance completed in 12 minutes and record it (in meters) on worksheet 8.1.

4. Use the regression equation below to predict $\dot{V}O_2$ max.

5. Compare the estimated $\dot{V}O_2$ max score to the norms listed in table 8.1.

Equation

$\dot{V}O_2$ max (mL $\cdot$ kg^{-1} $\cdot$ min^{-1}) = [0.0268 $\times$ distance in meters completed in 12 minutes] − 11.3

Sample Calculations

Gender: _Female_

Age: _22 years_

12-minute run distance: _1.1 miles_

Common conversion factors: 1.0 mile = 1,609.3 meters

1.0 yard = 0.9144 meter

1.0 foot = 0.3048 meter

Step 1: Convert distance in miles to meters.

1.1 miles $\times$ 1,609.3 meters = 1,770.2 meters completed in 12 minutes

Step 2: Calculate the predicted $\dot{V}O_2$max.

$\dot{V}O_2$ max = [0.0268 $\times$ 1,770.2] − 11.3 = 36.1 mL $\cdot$ kg^{-1} $\cdot$ min^{-1}

Step 3: Compare the predicted $\dot{V}O_2$ max score from the 12-minute run to the norms in table 8.1.

A score of 36.1 mL $\cdot$ kg^{-1} $\cdot$ min^{-1} would be classified as "good" for a 20- to 29-year-old woman in table 8.1.

| TABLE | 8.1 | Men's and women's aerobic fitness classification (predicted). |

MEN

Category	Measure	13–19	20–29	30–39	40–49	50–59	60+
				Age (years)			
I. Very Poor	$\dot{V}O_2$ max (mL • kg^{-1} • min^{-1})	<35.0	<33.0	<31.5	<30.2	<26.1	<20.5
II. Poor	$\dot{V}O_2$ max (mL • kg^{-1} • min^{-1})	35.0–38.3	33.0–36.4	31.5–35.4	30.2–33.5	26.1–30.9	20.5–26.0
III. Fair	$\dot{V}O_2$ max (mL • kg^{-1} • min^{-1})	38.4–45.1	36.5–42.4	35.5–40.9	33.6–38.9	31.0–35.7	26.1–32.2
IV. Good	$\dot{V}O_2$ max (mL • kg^{-1} • min^{-1})	45.2–50.9	42.5–46.4	41.0–44.9	39.0–43.7	35.8–40.9	32.2–36.4
V. Excellent	$\dot{V}O_2$ max (mL • kg^{-1} • min^{-1})	51.0–55.9	46.5–52.4	45.0–49.4	43.8–48.0	41.0–45.3	36.5–44.2
VI. Superior	$\dot{V}O_2$ max (mL • kg^{-1} • min^{-1})	>56.0	>52.5	>49.5	>48.1	>45.4	>44.3

WOMEN

Category	Measure	13–19	20–29	30–39	40–49	50–59	60+
				Age (years)			
I. Very Poor	$\dot{V}O_2$ max (mL • kg^{-1} • min^{-1})	<25.0	<23.6	<22.8	<21.0	<20.2	<17.5
II. Poor	$\dot{V}O_2$ max (mL • kg^{-1} • min^{-1})	25.0–30.9	23.6–28.9	22.8–26.9	21.0–24.4	20.2–22.7	17.5–20.1
III. Fair	$\dot{V}O_2$ max (mL • kg^{-1} • min^{-1})	31.0–34.9	29.0–32.9	27.0–31.4	24.5–28.9	22.8–26.9	20.2–24.4
IV. Good	$\dot{V}O_2$ max (mL • kg^{-1} • min^{-1})	35.0–38.9	33.0–36.9	31.50–35.6	29.0–32.8	27.0–31.4	24.5–30.2
V. Excellent	$\dot{V}O_2$ max (mL • kg^{-1} • min^{-1})	39.0–41.9	37.0–40.9	35.7–40.0	32.9–36.9	31.5–35.7	30.3–31.4
VI. Superior	$\dot{V}O_2$ max (mL • kg^{-1} • min^{-1})	>42.0	>41.0	>40.1	>37.0	>35.8	>31.5

Source: Cooper, Kenneth H. *The Aerobics Way.* Toronto: Bantam Books, 1977, pp. 280–281. Printed with permission of Kenneth H. Cooper, MD, MPH, www.cooperaerobics.com.

12-MINUTE RUN TEST FORM | Worksheet **8.1**

Name _____   Date _____

Gender: _____

1. Distance (in meters) completed in 12 minutes = _____

2. $\dot{V}O_2$ max (mL • kg^{-1} • min^{-1}) = [0.0268 × distance in meters completed in 12 minutes]
   − 11.3 = _____

3. Classification = _____ (see table 8.1)

EXTENSION ACTIVITIES | Worksheet **8.2**

Name _____   Date _____

Use the following data and table 8.1 to answer the questions below.

Gender: _____Male_____

Age: _____35 years_____

12-minute run distance: _____5,300 ft_____

1. Calculate the subject's predicted $\dot{V}O_2$max from the 12-minute run test.
   $\dot{V}O_2$ max = _____ (mL • kg^{-1} • min^{-1})

2. Classify the subject's predicted $\dot{V}O_2$max from the 12-minute run test (see table 8.1).
   Classification = _____

3. On the graph below, draw the expected relationship between the distance run in 12 minutes and $\dot{V}O_2$ max.

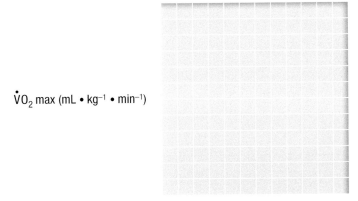

$\dot{V}O_2$ max (mL • kg^{-1} • min^{-1})

12-minute run distance

EXTENSION QUESTIONS

1. What are some common mistakes that may occur in administering this lab?

2. Identify possible sources of error in this lab.

3. Assess the practicality of using this lab in the field.

4. Research the reliability and/or validity of this lab using the Internet, journal articles, and other credible sources.

REFERENCES

1. Balke, B. A simple field test for the assessment of physical fitness. Report 63-6 Civil Aeromedical Research Institute. Oklahoma City: Federal Aviation Agency, 1963.

2. Cooper, K. H. A means of assessing maximal oxygen intake. *J. Am. Med. Assoc.* 203: 135–138, 1968.

3. Cramer, J. T., and Coburn, J. W. Fitness testing protocols and norms. In *NSCA's Essentials of Personal Training,* eds. R. W. Earle and T. R. Baechle. Champaign, IL: Human Kinetics, 2005, pp. 218–263.

4. Drinkard, B., McDuffie, J., McCann, S., Uwaifo, G. I., Nicholson, J., and Yanovski, J. A. Relationships between walk/run performance and cardiorespiratory fitness in adolescents who are overweight. *Phys. Ther.* 81: 1889–1896, 2001.

5. Heyward, V. H. *Advanced Fitness Assessment and Exercise Prescription,* 4th edition. Champaign, IL: Human Kinetics, 2002.

6. Jessup, G. T., Tolson, H., and Terry, J. W. Prediction of maximal oxygen intake from Astrand-Rhyming test, 12-minute run, and anthropometric variables using stepwise multiple regression. *Am. J. Phys. Med.* 53: 200–207, 1974.

7. McCutcheon, M. C., Sticha, S. A., Giese, M. D., and Nagle, F. J. A further analysis of the 12-minute run prediction of maximal aerobic power. *Res. Q. for Exerc. Sport.* 61: 280–283, 1990.

8. Safrit, M. J., Hooper, L. M., Ehlert, S. A., Costa, M. G., and Patterson, P. The validity generalization of distance run tests. *Can. J. Sport Sci.* 13: 188–196, 1988.

9. Wanamaker, G. S. A study of the validity and reliability of the 12-minute run under selected motivational conditions. *Am. Correct Ther. J.* 24: 69–72, 1970.

BACKGROUND

The 1.5-mile run test provides a simple method for estimating a person's maximal oxygen consumption rate ($\dot{V}O_2$ max) by measuring the elapsed time during 1.5 miles of running (or walking). Walking is allowed during this test; however, the objective is to complete the 1.5-mile distance as quickly as possible. A faster pace (speed) during the test will result in a lower time to complete the 1.5 miles, and, therefore, a higher predicted $\dot{V}O_2$ max. The following gender-specific regression equations have been developed[2] to predict $\dot{V}O_2$ max using body weight (kg) and the 1.5-mile run time (min):

MEN

$\dot{V}O_2$ max (mL $\bullet$ kg^{-1} $\bullet$ min^{-1}) = 91.736 $-$ (0.1656 $\times$ body weight in kg)
$-$ (2.767 $\times$ 1.5-mile run time in minutes)

R (multiple correlation coefficient) = 0.90

SEE (standard error of estimate) = 2.8 mL $\bullet$ kg^{-1} $\bullet$ min^{-1}

WOMEN

$\dot{V}O_2$ max (mL $\bullet$ kg^{-1} $\bullet$ min^{-1}) = 88.020 $-$ (0.1656 $\times$ body weight in kg)
$-$ (2.767 $\times$ 1.5-mile run time in minutes)

R (multiple correlation coefficient) = 0.90

SEE (standard error of estimate) = 2.8 mL $\bullet$ kg^{-1} $\bullet$ min^{-1}

The standard error of estimate values associated with these equations represents approximately 6.0% of $\dot{V}O_2$ max.

KNOW THESE TERMS & ABBREVIATIONS

☐ R = multiple correlation coefficient; a numerical measure of how well a dependent variable can be predicted from a combination of independent variables (a number between -1 and 1)

☐ SEE = standard error of estimate; a measure of the accuracy of the predictions made using a regression equation

☐ $\dot{V}O_2$ max = maximal oxygen consumption rate

EQUIPMENT (see Appendix 2 for vendors)   Approximate Price

1. A 400-meter track or a flat course that has been accurately measured for the distance of 1.5 miles (2.4 kilometers)
2. Scale $175
3. Stopwatch $10

PROCEDURES[3]

1. Measure body weight (in kilograms) on a scale.
2. Have the subject(s) warm up by walking and/or jogging for 5 minutes prior to the test.
3. Instruct the subject to run (or walk if necessary) as fast as possible for 1.5 miles (2.4 kilometers). Emphasize that a faster speed will result in a higher predicted $\dot{V}O_2$ max.
4. Measure the time it takes to complete the 1.5 miles and record it (in minutes) on worksheet 9.1.
5. Use one of the regression equations below to predict $\dot{V}O_2$ max.
6. Compare the estimated $\dot{V}O_2$ max score to the norms listed in table 9.1.

Equations

MEN

$\dot{V}O_2$ max (mL • kg^{-1} • min^{-1}) = 91.736 − (0.1656 × body mass in kg) − (2.767 × 1.5-mile run time in min)

WOMEN

$\dot{V}O_2$ max (mL • kg^{-1} • min^{-1}) = 88.020 − (0.1656 × body mass in kg) − (2.767 × 1.5-mile run time in min)

Sample Calculations

Gender: _Female_
Age: _28 years_
Body weight: _54 kg_
1.5-mile run time: _12:24 min:sec_

Step 1: Convert time to minutes.

24 sec ÷ 60 sec = 0.4 min

Therefore,

12:24 min:sec = 12.4 min

Step 2: Calculate the predicted $\dot{V}O_2$ max.

$\dot{V}O_2$ max = 88.020 − (0.1656 × 54 kg) − (2.767 × 12.4 min)
= 44.8 mL • kg^{-1} • min^{-1}

Step 3: Compare the predicted $\dot{V}O_2$ max score from the 12-minute run to the norms in table 9.1.

A score of 44.8 mL • kg^{-1} • min^{-1} would be classified as "superior" for a 20- to 29-year-old woman in table 9.1.

21 years
Time: 11:50 min sec

VO_2 max = 91.736 − (0.1656 × 65 kg) − (2.767 × 11.5)
31.82

VO_2 max = 91.736 − 10.764 − 31.82

Men's and women's aerobic fitness classification (predicted). **TABLE 9.1**

MEN							
		Age (years)					
Category	Measure	13–19	20–29	30–39	40–49	50–59	60+
I. Very Poor	$\dot{V}O_2$ max (mL • kg^{-1} • min^{-1})	<35.0	<33.0	<31.5	<30.2	<26.1	<20.5
II. Poor	$\dot{V}O_2$ max (mL • kg^{-1} • min^{-1})	35.0–38.3	33.0–36.4	31.5–35.4	30.2–33.5	26.1–30.9	20.5–26.0
III. Fair	$\dot{V}O_2$ max (mL • kg^{-1} • min^{-1})	38.4–45.1	36.5–42.4	35.5–40.9	33.6–38.9	31.0–35.7	26.1–32.2
IV. Good	$\dot{V}O_2$ max (mL • kg^{-1} • min^{-1})	45.2–50.9	42.5–46.4	41.0–44.9	39.0–43.7	35.8–40.9	32.2–36.4
V. Excellent	$\dot{V}O_2$ max (mL • kg^{-1} • min^{-1})	51.0–55.9	46.5–52.4	45.0–49.4	43.8–48.0	41.0–45.3	36.5–44.2
VI. Superior	$\dot{V}O_2$ max (mL • kg^{-1} • min^{-1})	>56.0	>52.5	>49.5	>48.1	>45.4	>44.3

WOMEN							
		Age (years)					
Category	Measure	13–19	20–29	30–39	40–49	50–59	60+
I. Very Poor	$\dot{V}O_2$ max (mL • kg^{-1} • min^{-1})	<25.0	<23.6	<22.8	<21.0	<20.2	<17.5
II. Poor	$\dot{V}O_2$ max (mL • kg^{-1} • min^{-1})	25.0–30.9	23.6–28.9	22.8–26.9	21.0–24.4	20.2–22.7	17.5–20.1
III. Fair	$\dot{V}O_2$ max (mL • kg^{-1} • min^{-1})	31.0–34.9	29.0–32.9	27.0–31.4	24.5–28.9	22.8–26.9	20.2–24.4
IV. Good	$\dot{V}O_2$ max (mL • kg^{-1} • min^{-1})	35.0–38.9	33.0–36.9	31.50–35.6	29.0–32.8	27.0–31.4	24.5–30.2
V. Excellent	$\dot{V}O_2$ max (mL • kg^{-1} • min^{-1})	39.0–41.9	37.0–40.9	35.7–40.0	32.9–36.9	31.5–35.7	30.3–31.4
VI. Superior	$\dot{V}O_2$ max (mL • kg^{-1} • min^{-1})	>42.0	>41.0	>40.1	>37.0	>35.8	>31.5

Source: Cooper, Kenneth H. *The Aerobics Way.* Toronto: Bantam Books, 1977, pp. 280–281. Printed with permission of Kenneth H. Cooper, MD, MPH, www.cooperaerobics.com.

$\dot{V}O_2$max = 49.15

Age – 20-29

Category – Excellent

Worksheet 9.1 | 1.5-MILE RUN TEST FORM

Name _____ Date _____

Gender: _____ *Male* _____

Age (years): _____ 21 _____

Body weight (kg): _____ 65 _____

1. Time (in min:sec) to complete the 1.5-mile run = minutes

2. Equation for men: $\dot{V}O_2$ max $(mL \cdot kg^{-1} \cdot min^{-1}) = 91.736 - (0.1656 \times$ body weight in kg$)$
   $- (2.767 \times$ 1.5-mile run time in min$) =$ _____ 32 _____

   Equation for women: $\dot{V}O_2$ max $(mL \cdot kg^{-1} \cdot min^{-1}) = 88.020 - (0.1656 \times$ body weight in kg$)$
   $- (2.767 \times$ 1.5-mile run time in min$) =$ _____ _____

3. Classification = _____ fair _____ (see table 9.1)

$91.736 - (0.1656 \times 65) - (2.767 \times 11.5$

$91.736 - 10.764 = 31.82$

32

Name _____   Date _____

Use the following data and table 9.1 to answer the questions below.

Gender: _____Male_____

Age: _____18 years_____

Body weight: _____82 kg_____

1.5-mile run time: _____13:45 min:sec_____

1. Calculate the subject's predicted $\dot{V}O_2$ max from the 1.5-mile run test.

    $\dot{V}O_2$ max = _____40.9_____ ($mL \cdot kg^{-1} \cdot min^{-1}$)

2. Classify the subject's predicted $\dot{V}O_2$ max from the 1.5-mile run test (see table 9.1).

    Classification = _____Excellent_____

3. On the graph below, draw the expected relationship between 1.5-mile run times and $\dot{V}O_2$ max.

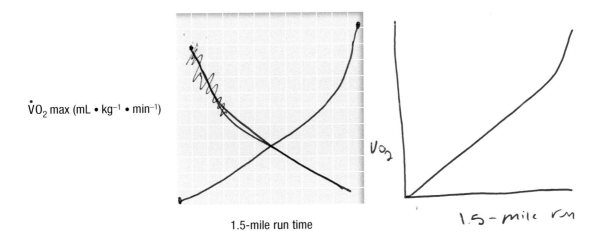

$\dot{V}O_2$ max ($mL \cdot kg^{-1} \cdot min^{-1}$)

1.5-mile run time

VO_2

1.5-mile rm

$$91.736 - (0.1656 \times 82) - 2.767 \times 13.45$$

$$40.9 \Rightarrow 41$$

EXTENSION QUESTIONS

1. What are some common mistakes that may occur in administering this lab?
2. Identify possible sources of error in this lab.
3. Assess the practicality of using this lab in the field.
4. Research the reliability and/or validity of this lab using the Internet, journal articles, and other credible sources.

REFERENCES

1. Cramer, J. T., and Coburn, J. W. Fitness testing protocols and norms. In *NSCA's Essentials of Personal Training,* eds. R. W. Earle and T. R. Baechle. Champaign, IL: Human Kinetics, 2005, pp. 218–263.
2. George, J. D., Vehrs, P. R., Allsen, P. E., Fellingham, G. W., and Fisher, A. G. VO₂max estimation from a submaximal 1-mile track jog for fit college-age individuals. *Med. Sci. Sports Exerc.* 81: 401–406, 1993.
3. Heyward, V. H. *Advanced Fitness Assessment and Exercise Prescription,* 4th edition. Champaign, IL: Human Kinetics, 2002.

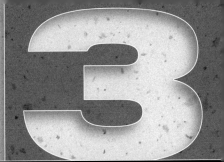

Unit 3

FATIGUE THRESHOLDS

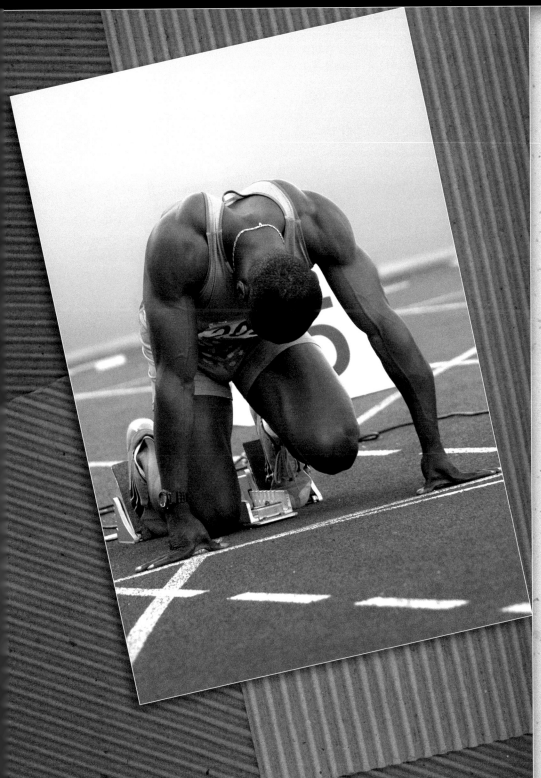

Non–Exercise-Based Estimation of the Ventilatory Threshold

BACKGROUND

Theoretically, the ventilatory threshold (VT) is an estimation of the exercise intensity above which anaerobic adenosine triphosphate (ATP) production must supplement aerobic metabolism. Thus, in theory, exercise intensities below the VT are non-fatiguing and are maintained from aerobic ATP production only, while those above the VT are fatiguing and utilize anaerobic plus aerobic ATP production. Typically, the VT occurs at approximately 50 to 60% of maximal oxygen consumption rate ($\dot{V}O_2$ max) in untrained to moderately trained individuals, but 80% of $\dot{V}O_2$ max or above in highly trained endurance athletes.[4]

The VT has been used as a measure of aerobic fitness in clinical populations including patients with HIV[6] and cystic fibrosis,[7] as well as endurance athletes such as marathon runners.[3,5] The VT has also been used to assess the effectiveness of endurance training programs.[1]

Endurance athletes with a high VT can maintain a high percentage (fraction) of their $\dot{V}O_2$ max for a long time without fatigue. Thus, an athlete with a high VT can maintain a faster race pace than a competitor with a lower VT and, therefore, perform better in endurance events. In fact, some elite distance runners with very high VT values can maintain a race pace that corresponds to approximately 90% of their $\dot{V}O_2$ max for the entire duration of a 26.2-mile marathon.

The VT is estimated from expired gas samples collected during an incremental test to exhaustion. During the test, the subjects breathes through a two-way valve to collect expired gas samples, which are then analyzed by a metabolic cart (see photo 10.1) to determine the volume of oxygen consumed ($\dot{V}O_2$ in L • min^{-1}) and the volume of carbon dioxide ($\dot{V}CO_2$ in L • min^{-1}) produced. As the exercise intensity increases, more oxygen is consumed per minute ($\dot{V}O_2$ increases) for ATP production, and a greater volume of carbon dioxide is produced ($\dot{V}CO_2$ increases). The $\dot{V}CO_2$ produced increases linearly with exercise intensity ($\dot{V}O_2$) until the VT is reached. Above the VT, there is a disproportionate increase in $\dot{V}CO_2$ (relative to $\dot{V}O_2$) as a result of the accelerated contribution of anaerobic energy to the metabolism. The VT is defined as the $\dot{V}O_2$ value (L • min^{-1}) that corresponds to the "breakpoint" (nonlinear increase) in the $\dot{V}CO_2$ versus $\dot{V}O_2$ relationship (see figure 10.1).

Direct determination of the VT in a laboratory setting requires a metabolic cart to analyze expired gas samples collected during the incremental test to

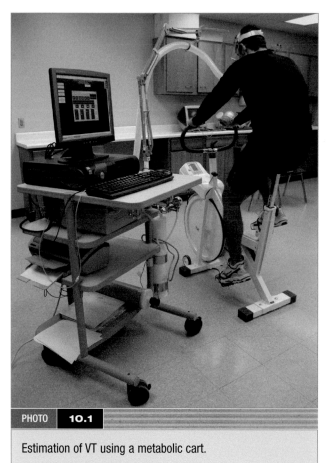

Estimation of VT using a metabolic cart.

Method for determining the ventilatory threshold (VT).   **FIGURE   10.1**

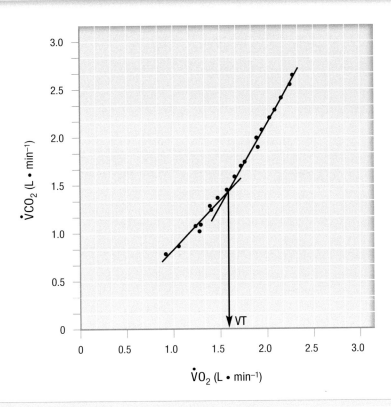

exhaustion. In this laboratory, however, the VT for adult males and females can be estimated using a multiple regression equation that utilizes only age and height as predictor variables.[2]

KNOW THESE TERMS & ABBREVIATIONS

- ☐ ATP = adenosine triphosphate
- ☐ $\dot{V}CO_2$ = the volume of CO_2 produced
- ☐ $\dot{V}O_2$ = oxygen consumption rate, an indirect measure of aerobic energy production
- ☐ $\dot{V}O_2$ max = maximal oxygen consumption rate
- ☐ VT = ventilatory threshold, an estimation of the exercise intensity above which anaerobic ATP production must supplement aerobic metabolism

EQUIPMENT (see Appendix 2 for vendors)   **Approximate Price**

Meter stick $10

PROCEDURES

1. Record the subject's age in years and height in cm (inches × 2.54) on worksheet 10.1.
2. Use the equation on the following page to calculate the VT.

Equation[2]

VT (L • min^{-1}) = (0.024 × height in cm) − (0.0074 × age in years) − 2.43

R (multiple correlation coefficient) = 0.651

SEE (standard error of estimate) = 0.316 L • min^{-1}

Note: This equation is used for both males and females.

Sample Calculation

Age: ___21___

Height: _70 inches (or 177.8 cm)_

VT (L • min^{-1}) = (0.024 × 177.8) − (0.0074 × 21) − 2.43 = 1.68 L • min^{-1}

| NON–EXERCISE-BASED ESTIMATION OF VENTILATORY THRESHOLD FORM | Worksheet **10.1** |

Name _____   Date _____

Age: _____21_____ yrs

Height: ~~14 73~~ cm
176.78

VT (L • min⁻¹) = (0.024 × height in cm) − (0.0074 × age in years) − 2.43 = ~~8948~~

4.0

$$0.024 \times 14.73 - 0.0074 \times 21$$

| EXTENSION ACTIVITIES | Worksheet **10.2** |

Name _____   Date _____

Use the following data to answer the questions below.

Age: 23 years

Height: 182 cm

$\dot{V}O_2$ max: 3.3 L • min⁻¹

1. Calculate the VT.

   VT = ____4.1____ L • min⁻¹

2. What percent of $\dot{V}O_2$ max is this VT value?

   VT = _____ % $\dot{V}O_2$ max

$$0.024 \times 182 - 0.0074 \times 23$$

EXTENSION QUESTIONS

1. What are some common mistakes that may occur in administering this lab?

2. Identify possible sources of error in this lab.

3. Assess the practicality of using this lab in the field.

4. Research the reliability and/or validity of this lab using the Internet, journal articles, and other credible sources.

REFERENCES

1. Jones, A. M., and Carter, H. The effects of endurance training on parameters of aerobic fitness. *Sports Med.* 29: 373–386, 2000.

2. Jones, N. L., Makrides, L., Hitchcock, C., Chypchar, T., and McCartney, N. Normal standards for an incremental progressive cycle ergometer test. *Am. Rev. Respir. Dis.* 131: 700–708, 1985.

3. Maffulli, N., Testa, V., and Gapasso, G. Anaerobic threshold determination in master endurance runners. *J. Sports Med. Phys. Fitness* 34: 242–249, 1994.

4. Malek, M. H., Housh, T. J., Coburn, J. W., Schmidt, R. J., and Beck, T. W. Cross-validation of ventilator threshold prediction equations on aerobically trained men and women. *J. Strength Cond. Res.* 21: 29–33, 2007.

5. Tanaka, K., and Matsuura, Y. Marathon performance, anaerobic threshold, and onset of blood lactate accumulation. *J. Appl. Physiol.* 57: 640–643, 1984.

6. Tesiorowski, A. M., Harris, M., Chan, K. J., Thompson, C. R., and Montaner, J. S. Anaerobic threshold and random venous lactate levels among HIV-positive patients on antiretroviral therapy. *J. Acquir. Immune Defic. Syndr.* 31: 250–251, 2002.

7. Thin, A. G., Linnane, S. J., McKone, E. F., Freaney R., Fitzgerald, M. X., Gallagher, C. G., and McLoughlin, P. Use of the gas exchange threshold to noninvasively determine the lactate threshold in patients with cystic fibrosis. *Chest* 121: 1761–1770, 2002.

BACKGROUND

Theoretically, the Critical Power (CP) cycle ergometer test estimates three parameters of physical working capacity:[1,2,3,4] (1) the maximal power output that can be maintained for an extended period of time without fatigue, called the CP; (2) the total amount of work that can be accomplished using only stored energy sources (creatine phosphate, glycogen, and oxygen bound to myoglobin) within the activated muscles, called the anaerobic work capacity (AWC); and (3) the time to exhaustion, or time limit (TL), during continuous cycle ergometry at any power output. The CP test uses linear mathematical modeling of the relationship between the total work accomplished at different power outputs and the corresponding TL values to simultaneously estimate the CP, AWC, and TL at any power output (figure 11.1).

Critical Power. The CP is an estimate of the maximal power output during cycle ergometry that can be maintained for an extended period of time without fatigue and is, conceptually, analogous to the anaerobic threshold.[4] The anaerobic threshold is one of three primary physiological factors (along with $\dot{V}O_2$max and economy of movement) that contribute to performance in endurance events. The anaerobic threshold is typically determined from the measurement of blood lactate levels (the lactate threshold) or expired gas samples (the ventilatory threshold). The CP, however, can be estimated using only a cycle ergometer and stopwatch and, therefore, does not require oxygen and carbon dioxide analyzers or invasive blood-sampling procedures.

Anaerobic Work Capacity. The AWC is an estimate of the total amount of work that can be accomplished using only stored energy sources within the activated muscles, such as creatine phosphate, glycogen, and oxygen bound to myoglobin.[1,4,5] Because it is not dependent upon the level of oxygen supply to the muscles,[4] the AWC represents anaerobic energy production capabilities, and it has been shown to be correlated with mean power from the Wingate Test[5] (see Lab 20). The ability to perform high-intensity, short-duration sports and activities such as weightlifting, 100–400 meter runs, 100–200 meter swims, gymnastics, basketball, football, and speed skating rely primarily on the anaerobic production of ATP to fuel muscle contraction. Thus, the CP test provides estimates of physical working capacity associated with both aerobic (the CP) and anaerobic (the AWC) ATP production.

Time to Exhaustion or Time Limit. There is a negative, curvilinear (asymptotic) relationship between power output and time to exhaustion that is called the power output versus TL curve (figure 11.1a). Based on his or her levels of aerobic and anaerobic fitness, each individual is characterized by a unique power output versus TL curve. That is, some individuals can maintain a particular power output for a long time, while other individuals fatigue rapidly at the same power output. The linear mathematical model used to estimate

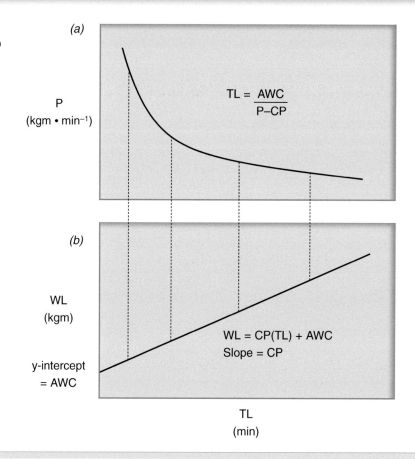

FIGURE 11.1 Curvilinear power output versus time limit relationship during cycle ergometry.

Figure 11.1a represents the negative, curvilinear power output (P) versus time limit (TL) relationship during cycle ergometry and provides the equation that can be used to estimate the TL for any P. Please note that, theoretically, any P ≤ CP can be maintained indefinitely without exhaustion. In reality, however, the CP can often be maintained for an extended period of time (usually > 30 minutes), but not indefinitely. Figure 11.1b represents the linear relationship between work limit (WL) and TL, and provides the equation that can be used to estimate the critical power (CP) and anaerobic work capacity (AWC).

CP and AWC (figure 11.1b) can also be used to derive an individual's power output versus TL curve and, therefore, estimate the time to exhaustion (TL) for any power output that is greater than the CP.[3] Theoretically, the CP is the asymptote of the power output versus TL relationship (figure 11.1a) and, therefore, any power output that is less than the CP should be able to be continued indefinitely. In reality, however, the CP can often be maintained for an extended period of time (usually > 30 minutes), but not indefinitely.[1,3]

KNOW THESE TERMS & ABBREVIATIONS

- ☐ ATP = adenosine triphosphate
- ☐ AWC = anaerobic work capacity (kgm), defined as the y-intercept of the work limit (WL) versus time limit (TL) relationship (figure 11.1b)
- ☐ CP = critical power (kgm • min⁻¹), defined as the slope coefficient of the work limit (WL) versus time limit (TL) relationship (figure 11.1b)
- ☐ P = power output (kgm • min⁻¹)
- ☐ TL = time limit (TL) or time to exhaustion (min)
- ☐ WL = work limit (WL) or total work performed (kgm)

EQUIPMENT (see Appendix 2 for vendors)   **Approximate Price**

1. Monark cycle ergometer $2,000
2. Stopwatch $10

PROCEDURES

The CP test will be performed using a Monark cycle ergometer and stop-watch. The three parameters of physical working capacity that will be determined are the CP, the AWC, and the TL for any power output. Use worksheet 11.1 to record the results of the CP test.

1. Prior to beginning the test: (1) adjust the seat height of the cycle ergometer to allow for near full extension of the subject's legs while pedaling and (2) record a pre-exercise heart rate.

2. Warm-up. The CP test will be preceded by a standardized warm-up protocol that includes four minutes of pedaling at 70 rpm and a resistance of 0.5 kg (power output = 210 kgm • min^{-1}).

3. Typically, the CP test involves a series of two or more cycle ergometer workbouts to exhaustion at different power outputs.[1,2,3,4,5] In this laboratory, two (or more) workbouts will be performed at a constant pedaling cadence of 70 rpm. The selection of power outputs for each subject usually ranges from approximately 1050 (2.5 kg resistance) to 2520 kgm • min^{-1} (6.0 kg resistance). See table 11.1. The power outputs should be selected so that the times to exhaustion (TL values in figure 11.1) for the shortest (highest power output) and longest (lowest power output) workbouts range from approximately one to 10 minutes and differ by five minutes or more.[1,2] For small and/or untrained

---

Resistance settings and corresponding power outputs at 70 rpm for a Monark cycle ergometer.   **TABLE**   **11.1**

Resistance (kg)	Power output (kgm • min^{-1})
1	420
1.5	630
2.0	840
2.5	1050
3.0	1260
3.5	1470
4.0	1680
4.5	1890
5.0	2100
5.5	2310
6.0	2520

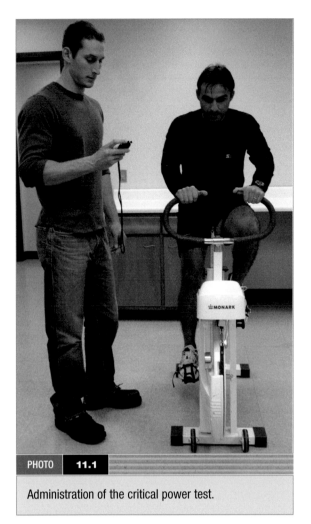

Administration of the critical power test.

subjects, the recommended power outputs when using only two workbouts for the CP test are 1260 kgm • min^{-1} (3.0 kg resistance) and 1680 kgm • min^{-1} (4.0 kg resistance). For large and/or trained subjects, as well as experienced cyclists, the recommended power outputs are 1470 kgm • min^{-1} (3.5 kg resistance) and 1890 kgm • min^{-1} (4.5 kg resistance). These power outputs should be viewed as only recommendations. It may be necessary to adjust them up or down to ensure that the subject's actual TL values are between approximately one and 10 minutes and differ by five minutes or more.[1,2]

4. Following the warm-up and a two-minute rest period, have the subject begin to pedal at 70 rpm and set the resistance (power output) to the appropriate level as quickly as possible during the first few seconds of the workbout. (See photo 11.1.)

5. Once the resistance is set, begin to time the workbout with a stopwatch.

6. Give the subject verbal encouragement to maintain the 70 rpm cadence for as long as possible. The workbout ends and the time to exhaustion is recorded when the subject can no longer maintain 65 rpm.[2,3] The subject must give an all-out effort to exhaustion during each workbout.

7. Cool-down. After each workbout, have the subject continue to pedal for two to three minutes (or longer if the subject desires) with no resistance.

8. No more than two workbouts at different power outputs should be performed on a single day. If a second workbout is to be performed during the same laboratory visit, have the subject rest (following the cool-down) until the person's heart rate returns to within 10 beats per minute of the pre-exercise level to ensure that he or she is fully recovered before performing the second workbout. This usually takes at least 30 minutes.[2,3]

Sample Calculations

Calculations of CP and AWC, as well as the derivation of the equation used to estimate the TL for any power output, follow.

1. Calculate the WL for each of the two (or more) workbouts by multiplying the imposed P (kgm • min^{-1}) by the TL (min).

FIRST WORKBOUT

P = 1680 kgm • min^{-1}

TL = 2 minutes and 20 seconds = 2.33 minutes

WL = 1680 × 2.33 = 3914 kgm

SECOND WORKBOUT

$P = 1260 \text{ kgm} \cdot \text{min}^{-1}$

TL = 7 minutes and 41 seconds = 7.68 minutes

WL = 1260 × 7.68 = 9677 kgm

2. Use a simple linear regression analysis (y = b(x) + a) to characterize the relationship for the WL (kgm) values for the two workbouts versus the corresponding TL values (figure 11.2b). Simple linear regression can be performed using many handheld calculators or software (such as Microsoft Excel and others) for PC and Macintosh computers. The slope coefficient and y-intercept values for the linear WL versus TL relationship are the CP and AWC, respectively (figure 11.2b).

	WL values	TL values
First workbout (1680 kgm · min⁻¹)	3914 kgm	2.33 minutes
Second workbout (1260 kgm · min⁻¹)	9677 kgm	7.68 minutes

Simple linear regression equation: WL = 1077(TL) + 1404

Thus,

$CP = 1077 \text{ kgm} \cdot \text{min}^{-1}$ and AWC = 1404 kgm

3. The linear regression analysis used to determine the CP and AWC for each subject is also used to derive the equation to estimate the TL for any P that is greater than CP (figure 11.2a). The equation is derived by equalizing the two mathematical expressions for determining the WL. That is,

WL = P(TL) = CP(TL) + AWC

Thus,

CP(TL) + AWC = P(TL)

AWC = P(TL) − CP(TL)

AWC = TL(P − CP)

$$\frac{AWC}{(P - CP)} = \frac{TL(P - CP)}{(P - CP)}$$

$$TL = \frac{AWC}{P - CP}$$

If a subject's CP = 1077 kgm · min⁻¹ and AWC = 1404 kgm, what is the estimated TL at a P of 2100 kgm · min⁻¹ (5.0 kg resistance)?

$$TL = \frac{1404}{2100 - 1077} = 1.37 \text{ minutes}$$

FIGURE   11.2   Graphic representations of sample calculations for CP (1077 kgm • min⁻¹), AWC (1404 kgm), and the estimated TL (1.37 min) at 2100 kgm • min⁻¹.

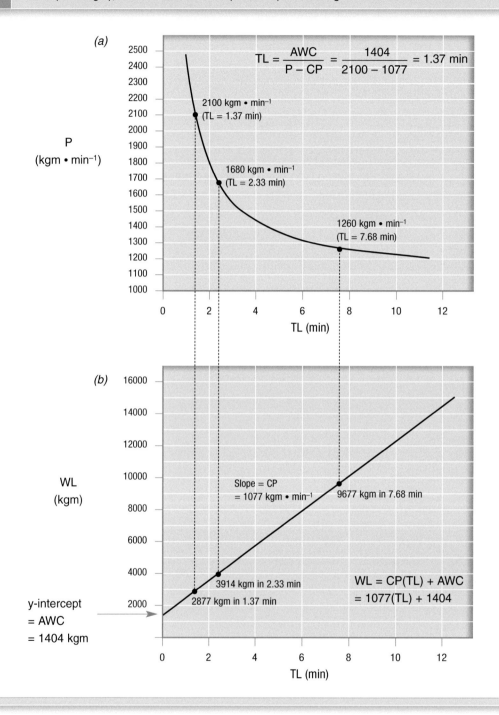

Name _____   Date _____

Seat height _____

Pre-exercise heart rate _____

Power Output (P)

Workbout 1: _____ kg of resistance $\times$ 420 [70 rpm (constant pedal cadence)]
$\times$ 6 meters (constant that defines the distance the flywheel travels each pedal revolution)]
= _____ kgm $\cdot$ min^{-1}

Workbout 2: _____ kg of resistance $\times$ 420 = _____ kgm $\cdot$ min^{-1}

Workbout 3 (if used): _____ kg of resistance $\times$ 420 = _____ kgm $\cdot$ min^{-1}

Workbout 4 (if used): _____ kg of resistance $\times$ 420 = _____ kgm $\cdot$ min^{-1}

Time Limit (TL)

Workbout 1: _____ min

Workbout 2: _____ min

Workbout 3: _____ min

Workbout 4: _____ min

Work Limit (WL)

Workbout 1: P _____ (kgm $\cdot$ min^{-1}) $\times$ TL _____ (min) = WL _____ kgm

Workbout 2: P _____ $\times$ TL _____ = WL _____ kgm

Workbout 3: P _____ $\times$ TL _____ = WL _____ kgm

Workbout 4: P _____ $\times$ TL _____ = WL _____ kgm

WL vs. TL Relationship

Use linear regression analysis to determine the equation that describes the WL vs. TL relationship:
WL = CP(TL) + AWC (see figure 11.2b).

CP = _____ kgm $\cdot$ min^{-1}

AWC = _____ kgm

$TL = \dfrac{AWC}{P - CP} = $ _____

Name _____ *Date* _____

1. A CP test resulted in the following data:

WL (kgm)	P	TL
8500	_____	_____
4500	_____	_____
2700	_____	_____
12000	_____	_____

Given the expected relationships among WL, P, and TL, fill in the blanks with the P and TL values from the randomly ordered choices below.

P (kgm • min^{-1}) = 1260, 1680, 1890, and 2310

TL (min) = 2.38, 1.17, 9.52, and 5.06

2. Given a CP of 1550 kgm • min^{-1} and an AWC of 1900 kgm, what is the estimated TL for a P of 1890 kgm • min^{-1}?

3. Use your own data to calculate the following:
   a. CP = _____ kgm • min^{-1}
   b. AWC = _____ kgm
   c. TL at a P of CP + 200 kgm • min^{-1} = _____ min

EXTENSION QUESTIONS

1. What are some common mistakes that may occur in administering this lab?
2. Identify possible sources of error in this lab.
3. Assess the practicality of using this lab in the field.
4. Research the reliability and/or validity of this lab using the Internet, journal articles, and other credible sources.

REFERENCES

1. Hill, D. W. The critical power concept. *Sports Med.* 4: 237–254, 1993.
2. Housh, D. J., Housh, T. J., and Bauge, S. M. A methodological consideration for the determination of critical power and anaerobic work capacity. *Res. Q. Exerc. Sport* 61: 406–409, 1990.
3. Housh, D. J., Housh, T. J., and Bauge, S. M. The accuracy of the critical power test for predicting time to exhaustion during cycle ergometry. *Ergonomics* 32: 997–1004, 1989.
4. Moritani, T., Nagata, A., deVries, H. A., and Muro, M. Critical power as a measure of physical work capacity and anaerobic threshold. *Ergonomics* 24: 339–350, 1981.
5. Nebelsick-Gullett, L. J., Housh, T. J., Johnson, G. O., and Bauge, S. M. A comparison between methods of measuring anaerobic work capacity. *Ergonomics* 31: 1413–1419, 1988.

Critical Velocity for Track Running Test

BACKGROUND

The purpose of this lab is to describe the procedures for performing the Critical Velocity (CV) test on a running track. The CV test estimates three parameters of physical working capacity:[1,2,3,4,5] (1) the maximal running velocity that can be maintained for an extended period of time without fatigue, called the CV; (2) the total distance that can be run using only stored energy sources (creatine phosphate, glycogen, and oxygen bound to myoglobin) within the activated muscles, called the anaerobic running capacity (ARC); and (3) the time to exhaustion or time limit (TL) during continuous running at any velocity (V). The CV test uses linear mathematical modeling of the relationship between the total distance (TD) at different velocities and the corresponding TL values to estimate the CV, ARC, and TL simultaneously at any velocity (Figure 12.1).

Critical Velocity (CV). The CV is an estimate of the maximal running velocity that can be maintained for an extended period of time without fatigue and is conceptually analogous to the anaerobic threshold.[2,4] The anaerobic threshold is one of three primary physiological factors (along with $\dot{V}O_2$max and economy of movement) that contribute to performance in endurance events. The anaerobic threshold is typically determined from the measurement of blood lactate levels (the lactate threshold) or expired gas samples (the ventilatory threshold). A salient feature of the critical velocity for track running test, however, is that it requires only a running track, markers (e.g., orange cones, reflective tape) placed at 100-meter intervals around the track, and a stopwatch.

Anaerobic Running Capacity (ARC). The ARC is an estimate of the total distance that can be run using only stored energy sources within the activated muscles, such as creatine phosphate, glycogen, and oxygen bound to myoglobin.[3] Theoretically, the ARC represents the capacity to produce ATP from anaerobic metabolic pathways. Thus, the CV test provides estimates of physical working capacity associated with both aerobic (the CV) and anaerobic (ARC) ATP production.

Time to Exhaustion or Time Limit (TL). There is a negative, curvilinear (asymptotic) relationship between V and TL that is called the V versus TL curve (figure 12.1a). Based on his or her fitness level, each individual has a unique V versus TL curve. The linear mathematical model used to estimate CV and ARC (Figure 12.1b) can also be used to derive an individual's V versus TL curve and, therefore, an equation to predict the person's TL for any V that is greater than the CV. Theoretically, the CV is the asymptote of the V versus TL curve (figure 12.1a) and, thus, any V ≤ CV should be able to be continued indefinitely. In reality, however, the CV can often be maintained for an extended period of time (usually > 30 minutes), but not indefinitely.[2,4,5]

Curvilinear velocity (V) versus time limit (TL) relationship.   FIGURE   12.1

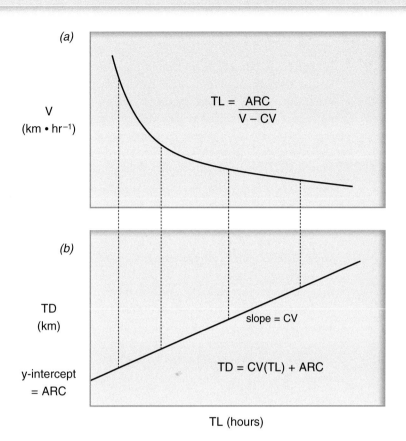

(a)

$$V$$
$$(km \cdot hr^{-1})$$

$$TL = \frac{ARC}{V - CV}$$

(b)

TD
(km)

slope = CV

$$TD = CV(TL) + ARC$$

y-intercept
= ARC

TL (hours)

Figure 12.1a represents the negative, curvilinear velocity (V) versus time limit (TL) relationship and provides the equation that can be used to estimate the TL for any V. Please note that, theoretically, any V less than the critical velocity (CV) can be maintained indefinitely without exhaustion. In reality, however, the CV can often be maintained for an extended period of time (usually > 30 minutes), but not indefinitely. Figure 12.1b represents the linear relationship between total distance (TD) and TL, and provides the equation that can be used to estimate the CV and anaerobic running capacity (ARC).

KNOW THESE TERMS & ABBREVIATIONS

☐ ARC = anaerobic running capacity (km), defined as the y-intercept of the total distance (TD) versus TL relationship (figure 12.1b)

☐ CV = critical velocity (km • hr^{-1}), defined as the slope coefficient of the total distance (TD) versus TL relationship (figure 12.1b).

☐ TL = time to exhaustion or time limit (TL) (hours)

☐ V = velocity (km • hr^{-1})

EQUIPMENT (see Appendix 2 for vendors)   **Approximate Price**

1. A 200- or 400-meter track or premeasured flat course

2. Markers (e.g., orange cones) $10

3. Stopwatch $10

PROCEDURES (See photo 12.1)

The CV test can be performed on either a 400-meter or a 200-meter track (or other length tracks with appropriate modifications for time splits). The equipment required for the test includes stopwatches and two or four markers that will be placed at 100-meter increments around the track. Four markers are

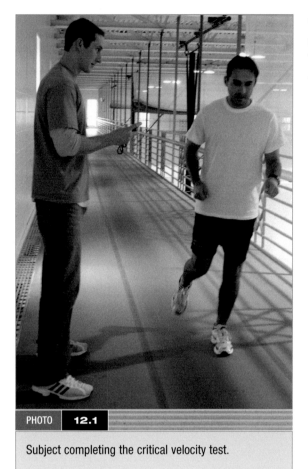

PHOTO **12.1**

Subject completing the critical velocity test.

used for a 400-meter track, and two markers are used for a 200-meter track. The three parameters of physical working capacity that will be determined are the CV, ARC, and TL for any V.

1. As stated previously, an important feature of the CV test is that it uses very little equipment. The test does, however, require two (or more) exhaustive runs, each of which is performed at a different constant velocity. To achieve constant velocities during the runs, the subjects will be required to reach 100-meter intervals on the track at designated time points, or splits. For example, with a 400-meter track, four markers are placed at 100-meter intervals around the track. If a subject is required to run at a velocity of 18 km • hr^{-1} (11.18 mph), he or she should reach the first marker (i.e., 100 meters away from the starting line) in 20 seconds, the second marker in 40 seconds, the third marker in 60 seconds, and the starting line in 80 seconds (figure 12.2). Figure 12.2 shows the 100-meter time splits required for four different velocities. It is important to note that the same time splits can be used for a 200-meter track. With a 200-meter track, however, only two markers (one at the starting line and another one 100 meters away from the starting line) are used. For untrained subjects, the recommended 100-meter time splits when using only two runs for the CV test are 30 seconds (12 km • hr^{-1} or 7.45 mph) and 20 seconds (18 km • hr^{-1} or 11.18 mph). For trained subjects or experienced runners, the recommended 100-meter time splits are 25 seconds (14.4 km • hr^{-1} or 8.94 mph) and 15 seconds (24 km • hr^{-1} or 14.91 mph).

2. Warm-up. Prior to the warm-up, record a pre-exercise heart rate. The CV test should be preceded by a warm-up that includes three minutes of walking and then three minutes of jogging at a comfortable pace around the track.

3. Following the warm-up and a two-minute rest period, instruct the subject that during the test, he or she should run at the designated time splits for as long as possible. The run ends when the subject cannot maintain the designated split time.

4. When the subject is ready to begin the test, have him or her start a stopwatch and run toward the first marker to complete the first time split. If the subject is unable to accomplish any of the first four time splits, he or she should stop the test and rest until his or her heart rate is within 10 beats per minute of the resting heart rate. The test should then be restarted at a lower velocity.

5. For each run, the TL is recorded on worksheet 12.1 when the subject can no longer complete the designated time splits. The TL is then calculated with the following equation:

TL = number of time splits (each 100 meters) successfully completed
× duration (in seconds) of each split

Example of the marker locations for the critical velocity (CV) test with a 400-meter track.   **FIGURE   12.2**

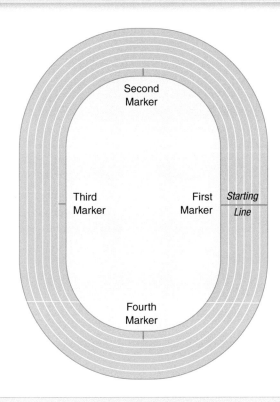

The 100-meter time splits are shown. Note that the CV test can also be performed with a 200-meter track, in which case only two markers would be used (one at the starting line, and another one that is 100 meters away from the starting line).

100-meter time splits for four running velocities

15-second time splits = 24 km • hr^{-1} or 14.91 mph

20-second time splits = 18 km • hr^{-1} or 11.18 mph

25-second time splits = 14.4 km • hr^{-1} or 8.94 mph

30-second time splits = 12 km • hr^{-1} or 7.45 mph

For example, if the subject ran 20-second time splits and was able to complete eight splits, then the TL was 160 seconds (8 time splits × 20 seconds per split), or 0.044 hours. The corresponding TD can then be calculated with the following equation:

TD = number of time splits successfully completed × distance (in meters) of each split

Thus, the TD for this example would be 800 meters (8 time splits × 100 meters per split), or 0.8 km.

6. Cool-down. After each exhaustive run, have the subject walk around the track at a comfortable pace for as long as desired.

7. No more than two exhaustive runs at different velocities (time splits) should be performed on a single day. If a second run is to be performed on the same day, have the subject rest (following the cool-down) until his or her heart rate returns to within 10 beats per minute of the pre-exercise level to ensure that the individual is fully recovered before performing the second run. This usually takes at least 30 minutes.

Sample Calculations

Calculations of CV and ARC, as well as the derivation of the equation used to estimate the TL for any V, follow.

1. Calculate the TL and TD for each of the two or more track runs at different velocities.

FIRST RUN

100 meter time split = 20 seconds (18 km • hr^{-1})

Number of time splits successfully completed = 8

TL = 8 time splits × 20 seconds per split = 160 seconds = 0.044 hours

TD = 8 time splits × 100 meters per split = 800 meters = 0.8 km

SECOND RUN

100 meter time split = 30 seconds (12 km • hr^{-1})

Number of time splits successfully completed = 14

TL = 14 time splits × 30 seconds per split = 420 seconds = 0.117 hours

TD = 14 time splits × 100 meters per split = 1400 meters = 1.4 km

2. Use a simple linear regression analysis (y = b(x) + a) to characterize the relationship for the TD (km) values for the two track runs versus the corresponding TL (hours) values (figure 12.3b). Simple linear regression can be performed using many handheld calculators or software (such as Microsoft Excel and others) for PC and Macintosh computers. The slope coefficient and y-intercept values for the linear TD versus TL relationship are the CV and ARC, respectively (figure 12.3b).

	TD (km)	TL (hours)
First run (20-second time splits)	0.8	0.044
Second run (30-second time splits)	1.4	0.117

Simple linear regression equation: TD = 8.22(TL) + 0.44

Thus,

CV = 8.22 km • hr^{-1} and ARC = 0.44 km.

3. The linear regression analysis used to determine the CV and ARC for each subject is also used to derive the equation to estimate the TL for any velocity that is greater than CV (figure 12.3a). The equation is derived by equalizing the two mathematical expressions for determining the TD. That is,

TD = V(TL) = CV(TL) + ARC

Thus,

CV(TL) + ARC = V(TL)

ARC = V(TL) − CV(TL)

ARC = TL(V − CV)

$$\frac{ARC}{(V - CV)} = \frac{TL(V - CV)}{(V - CV)}$$

$$TL = \frac{ARC}{V - CV}$$

If a subject's CV = 8.22 km • hr^{-1} and ARC = 0.44 km, what is his or her TL at a velocity of 16 km • hr^{-1}?

$$TL = \frac{0.44}{16 - 8.22} = 0.057 \text{ hours (3.42 minutes)}$$

Graphic representation of sample calculations for critical velocity (CV = 8.22 km • hr⁻¹), anaerobic running capacity (ARC = 0.44 km), and the estimated time limit (TL = 0.057 hours) at 16 km • hr⁻¹.

FIGURE **12.3**

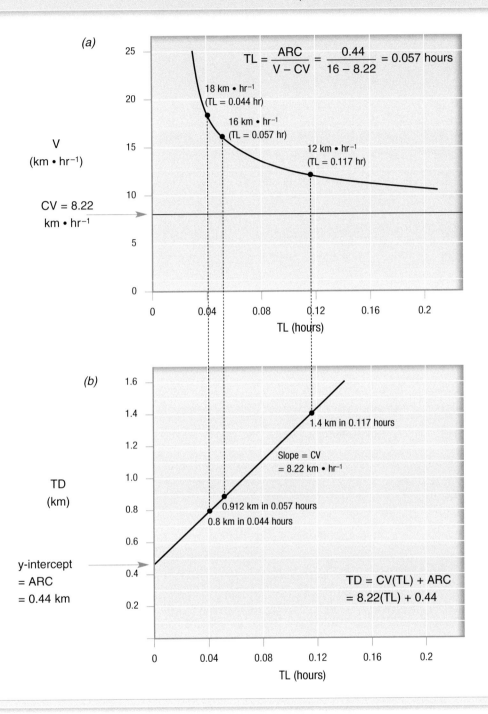

Worksheet 12.1 | CRITICAL VELOCITY FOR TRACK RUNNING TEST FORM

Name _____   Date _____

Pre-exercise Heart Rate _____

Velocity (V)   *Time splits*

Velocity 1: _____ km • hr^{-1} _____ sec

Velocity 2: _____ km • hr^{-1} _____ sec

Velocity 3 (if used): _____ km • hr^{-1} _____ sec

Velocity 4 (if used): _____ km • hr^{-1} _____ sec

Time Limit (TL)

Velocity 1: Number of splits completed ____ × ____ seconds per split = ____ seconds ÷ 3600 = ____ hours

Velocity 2: Number of splits completed ____ × ____ seconds per split = ____ seconds ÷ 3600 = ____ hours

Velocity 3: Number of splits completed ____ × ____ seconds per split = ____ seconds ÷ 3600 = ____ hours

Velocity 4: Number of splits completed ____ × ____ seconds per split = ____ seconds ÷ 3600 = ____ hours

Total Distance (TD)

Velocity 1: Number of splits completed ____ × 100 meters per split = ____ m ÷ 1000 = ____ km

Velocity 2: Number of splits completed ____ × 100 meters per split = ____ m ÷ 1000 = ____ km

Velocity 3: Number of splits completed ____ × 100 meters per split = ____ m ÷ 1000 = ____ km

Velocity 4: Number of splits completed ____ × 100 meters per split = ____ m ÷ 1000 = ____ km

TD vs. TL Relationship

Use linear regression analysis to determine the equation that describes the TD vs. TL relationship:
TD = CV(TL) + ARC (see figure 12.3b)

CV = _____ km • hr^{-1}

ARC = _____ km

Equation for estimating the TL at any V (see figure 12.3a)

$$TL = \frac{ARC}{V - CV} = \text{_____ hours}$$

Name _____   Date _____

1. A critical velocity for track running test resulted in the following data:

TD (km)	V (km • hr⁻¹)	TL (hours)
2.64	_____	_____
2.32	_____	_____
1.20	_____	_____
1.12	_____	_____

Given the expected relationships among TD, V, and TL, fill in the blanks with the V and TL values from the randomly ordered choices below.

   V (km • hr⁻¹) = 18.5, 16.9, 19.3, 17.7

   TL (hours) = 0.065, 0.058, 0.131, 0.156

2. Given a CV of 15.94 km • hr⁻¹ and an ARC of 0.19 km, what is the estimated TL for a V of 18.0 km • hr⁻¹?

3. Use your own data to calculate the following:

   a. CV = _____ km • hr⁻¹

   b. ARC = _____ km

   c. TL at a V of CV + 2.0 km • hr⁻¹ = _____ hours

EXTENSION QUESTIONS

1. What are some common mistakes that may occur in administering this lab?
2. Identify possible sources of error in this lab.
3. Assess the practicality of using this lab in the field.
4. Research the reliability and/or validity of this lab using the Internet, journal articles, and other credible sources.

REFERENCES

1. Housh, T. J., Cramer, J. T., Bull, A. J., Johnson, G. O., and Housh, D. J. The effect of mathematical modeling on critical velocity. *Eur. J. Appl. Physiol.* 84: 469–475, 2001.

2. Housh, T. J., Johnson, G. O., McDowell, S. L., Housh, D. J., and Pepper, M. Physiological responses at the fatigue threshold. *Int. J. Sports Med.* 12: 305–308, 1991.

3. Housh, T. J., Johnson, G. O., McDowell, S. L., Housh, D. J., and Pepper, M. The relationship between anaerobic running capacity and peak plasma lactate. *J. Sports Med. Phys. Fitness* 32: 117–122, 1992.

4. Hughson, R. L., Orok, C. J., and Staudt, L. E. A high velocity treadmill running test to assess endurance running potential. *Int. J. Sports Med.* 5: 23–25, 1984.

5. Pepper, M. L., Housh, T. J., and Johnson, G. O. The accuracy of the critical velocity test for predicting time to exhaustion during treadmill running. *Int. J. Sports Med.* 13: 121–124, 1992.

BACKGROUND

Theoretically, the physical working capacity at the heart rate threshold (PWC_{HRT}) test provides an estimate of the maximal power output during cycle ergometry that can be maintained for a very long period of time (four to eight hours) with no increase in heart rate (e.g., a steady-state heart rate).[1,2] The PWC_{HRT} test is most applicable to situations where assessing the ability to perform long-term, submaximal physical activity is more important than defining a subject's maximal exercise capacity (such as maximal oxygen consumption rate, $\dot{V}O_2$ max). Potential applications of the PWC_{HRT} test include assessing the physical working capacity of workers in industrial settings where strenuous labor is performed for eight or more hours per day, evaluating the effectiveness of endurance-training programs in a variety of populations including the elderly, and examining the training status of ultra-endurance athletes such as triathletes or long-distance cyclists.[1,3] Furthermore, the submaximal protocol used to determine the PWC_{HRT} makes it appropriate for assessing aerobic fitness in subjects where maximal exercise testing may be contraindicated, such as the elderly or clinical populations.

The PWC_{HRT} test involves performing two or more eight-minute workouts at different submaximal power outputs. This lab will describe the procedures for estimating the PWC_{HRT} using two workouts performed on the same day. Three or four workouts, however, can also be used if the PWC_{HRT} test is completed over two or more days. During each workout, heart rate (HR) is recorded and the slope coefficient for the HR versus time relationship is determined. The power output values are then plotted as a function of the slope coefficients for the HR versus time relationships, and the y-intercept is defined as the PWC_{HRT} (see figure 13.1b, page 89). Salient features of the PWC_{HRT} test are that it requires only submaximal exercise, and it can be performed using only a cycle ergometer, stopwatch, and heart rate monitoring system.

KNOW THESE TERMS & ABBREVIATIONS

☐ HR = heart rate (bpm)

☐ PWC_{HRT} = physical working capacity at the heart rate threshold (watts), defined as the y-intercept of the power output versus HR slope coefficient relationship (figure 13.1b)

☐ $\dot{V}O_2$max = maximal oxygen consumption rate

EQUIPMENT (see Appendix 2 for vendors)	**Approximate Price**
1. Monark cycle ergometer	$2,000
2. Heart rate monitor	$100
3. Stopwatch	$10

PROCEDURES (See photos 13.1 and 13.2)

The PWC$_{HRT}$ test will be performed using a Monark cycle ergometer, heart rate monitoring system, and stopwatch.

1. Prior to beginning the test: (1) adjust the seat height of the cycle ergometer to allow for near full extension of the subject's legs while pedaling, (2) fit the subject with a heart rate monitoring system (see photo 13.1), and (3) record a pre-exercise heart rate (see photo 13.2).

2. Warm-up: The PWC$_{HRT}$ test should be preceded by a standardized warm-up protocol that includes four minutes of pedaling at 70 rpm at a resistance of 0.5 kg (power output = 34 watts).

3. The PWC$_{HRT}$ test involves two to four cycle ergometer workbouts at different power outputs.[1,2,3] Each workbout is performed at a constant pedaling cadence of 70 rpm, and the selection of power outputs for each subject usually ranges from approximately 52 (0.75 kg resistance) to 223 (3.25 kg resistance) watts.[2,3] See table 13.1. The power outputs should be selected low enough so that the subject is able to complete the full eight minutes for each workbout, but high enough to elicit a positive slope in the HR versus time relationship. Record the selected power outputs on worksheet 13.1. For small or untrained subjects, the recommended power outputs for the PWC$_{HRT}$ test are between 52 (0.75 kg resistance) and 137 (2.0 kg resistance) watts. For large or trained subjects, as well as experienced cyclists, the recommended power outputs are between 137 (2.0 kg resistance) and 223 (3.25 kg resistance) watts. These power outputs, however, should be viewed as only recommendations. It may be necessary to adjust them up or down to ensure that the HR versus time slope coefficient is positive and the subject is able to complete the entire eight-minute workbout.

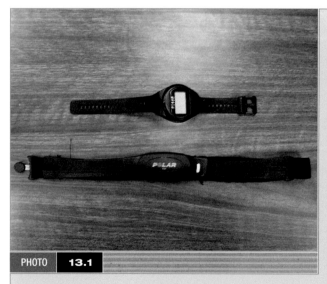

PHOTO 13.1

A heart rate monitoring system.

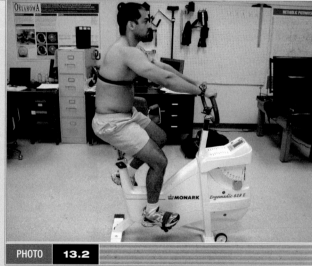

PHOTO 13.2

Positioning of the subject on the cycle ergometer for recording the pre-exercise heart rate.

4. Following the warm-up and a two-minute rest period, have the subject begin to pedal at 70 rpm, and set the resistance (power output) to the appropriate level as quickly as possible during the first few seconds of the workbout.

5. Once the resistance is set, begin to time the workbout with a stopwatch.

6. Give the subject verbal encouragement to maintain the 70 rpm cadence. Record a HR on worksheet 13.1 at the end of minutes 3, 4, 5, 6, and 7. HR data should not be collected during the first three minutes to allow for the initial cardiac adjustment to exercise.

7. Cool-down. After each workbout, allow the subject to continue to pedal for two to three minutes (or longer if the subject desires) with no resistance.

8. The two workbouts at different power outputs can be performed on a single day. If a second workbout is to be performed during the same laboratory visit, have the subject rest (following the cool-down) until the heart rate returns to within 10 beats per minute of the pre-exercise level to ensure that the individual is fully recovered before performing the second workbout. This usually takes at least 30 minutes.

Resistance settings and corresponding power outputs at 70 rpm for a Monark cycle ergometer.   **TABLE**   **13.1**

Resistance (kg)	Power output (watts)
0.50	34
0.75	52
1.00	69
1.25	86
1.50	103
1.75	120
2.00	137
2.25	154
2.50	172
2.75	189
3.00	206
3.25	223
3.50	240
3.75	257
4.00	275

Sample Calculations

1. Use simple linear regression analysis (y = b(x) + a) to calculate the slope coefficient for the HR versus time relationship for each workbout (figure 13.1a). Simple linear regression can be performed using many handheld calculators or software (such as Microsoft Excel and others) for PC and Macintosh computers.

TIME (min)	WORKBOUT 1 HR (bpm)	WORKBOUT 2 HR (bpm)
1	HR data not recorded to allow for the	
2	initial cardiac adjustment to exercise	
3	↓	↓
4	138	154
5	140	158
6	143	163
7	146	166
8	149	172

For workbout 1, enter the x-values as 4, 5, 6, 7, and 8, and the y-values as 138, 140, 143, 146, and 149.

Workbout 1 simple linear regression equation: HR = 2.8 (time) + 126.4

Thus, workbout 1 HR versus time slope coefficient = 2.8 bpm • min^{-1}

For workbout 2, enter the x-values as 4, 5, 6, 7, and 8, and the y-values as 154, 158, 163, 166, and 172.

Workbout 2 simple linear regression equation: HR = 4.4(time) + 136.2

Thus, workbout 2 HR versus time slope coefficient = 4.4 bpm • min^{-1}

2. Use simple linear regression analysis (y = b(x) + a) to calculate the y-intercept (i.e., the PWC_{HRT}) for the power output versus HR slope coefficient relationship (figure 13.1b).

	HR versus time slope coefficient (bpm • min^{-1})	Power output (watts)
Workbout 1	2.8	125
Workbout 2	4.4	175

Simple linear regression equation: Power output = 31.3 (HR versus time slope coefficient) + 37.5.

Thus, the estimated maximal power output that can be maintained with no change in HR over time (PWC_{HRT}) = 37.5 watts.

Description of the method for estimating the physical working capacity at the heart rate threshold (PWC$_{HRT}$).

FIGURE   13.1

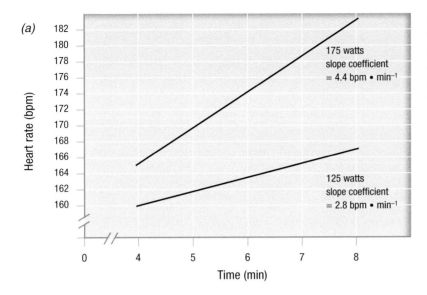

(a)

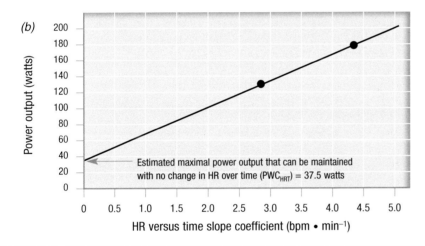

(b)

(a) The heart rate (HR) data are plotted as a function of time for various power outputs on a cycle ergometer. (b) The slope coefficients from (a) are plotted for each of the power outputs, and the PWC$_{HRT}$ is estimated as the y-intercept value.

Worksheet **13.1**	**PHYSICAL WORKING CAPACITY AT THE HEART RATE THRESHOLD (PWC$_{HRT}$) TEST FORM**

Name _____   *Date* _____

Seat height _____

Pre-exercise heart rate _____ bpm

Power Output

Workbout 1: _____ kg of resistance × 420 [70 rpm (constant pedal cadence) × 6 meters (constant that defines the distance the flywheel travels each pedal revolution)] / 6.12 = _____ watts

Workbout 2: _____ kg of resistance × 420 / 6.12 = _____ watts

Workbout 3 (if used): _____ kg of resistance × 420 / 6.12 = _____ watts

Workbout 4 (if used): _____ kg of resistance × 420 / 6.12 = _____ watts

Time (min)	Workbout 1 HR (bpm)	Workbout 2 HR (bpm)	Workbout 3 HR (bpm)	Workbout 4 HR (bpm)
1	Do not collect HR data for the first three minutes to allow for the initial cardiac adjustment to exercise.			
2				
3				
4	_____	_____	_____	_____
5	_____	_____	_____	_____
6	_____	_____	_____	_____
7	_____	_____	_____	_____
8	_____	_____	_____	_____

HR Versus Time Slope Coefficient

Use linear regression analysis to determine the slope coefficient for the HR versus time relationship for each workbout: $y = b(x) + a$

    Workbout 1: _____ bpm • min^{-1}

    Workbout 2: _____ bpm • min^{-1}

    Workbout 3 (if used): _____ bpm • min^{-1}

    Workbout 4 (if used): _____ bpm • min^{-1}

Use linear regression analysis to determine the y-intercept (i.e., PWC$_{HRT}$) of the power output versus HR slope coefficient relationship:

    Power output = b(HR slope coefficient) + PWC$_{HRT}$ (See figure 13.1b).

    PWC$_{HRT}$ = _____ watts

Name   *Date*

1. Two subjects performed four separate eight-minute workbouts on a cycle ergometer at the following power outputs: workbout 1 = 125 watts, workbout 2 = 150 watts, workbout 3 = 175 watts, and workbout 4 = 200 watts. The HR responses for each subject and workbout are shown below:

SUBJECT A

Time (min)	Workbout 1 HR (bpm)	Workbout 2 HR (bpm)	Workbout 3 HR (bpm)	Workbout 4 HR (bpm)
4	137	140	154	163
5	140	143	158	167
6	142	146	163	173
7	146	150	168	179
8	148	153	172	184

SUBJECT B

Time (min)	Workbout 1 HR (bpm)	Workbout 2 HR (bpm)	Workbout 3 HR (bpm)	Workbout 4 HR (bpm)
4	155	163	169	170
5	159	168	174	175
6	161	172	181	182
7	164	177	188	188
8	168	183	193	196

Which subject has the higher PWC$_{HRT}$? subject A or subject B (circle the correct choice)

2. Describe two advantages of the PWC$_{HRT}$ test when compared to a $\dot{V}O_2$max test.

3. Use your own data to calculate your PWC$_{HRT}$.

EXTENSION QUESTIONS

1. What are some common mistakes that may occur in administering this lab?

2. Identify possible sources of error in this lab.

3. Assess the practicality of using this lab in the field.

4. Research the reliability and/or validity of this lab using the Internet, journal articles, and other credible sources.

REFERENCES

1. Perry, S. R., Housh, T. J., Johnson, G. O., Ebersole, K. T., and Bull, A. J. Heart rate and ratings of perceived exertion at the physical working capacity at the heart rate threshold. *J. Strength Cond. Res.* 15: 225–229, 2001.

2. Wagner, L. L., and Housh, T. J. A proposed test for determining physical working capacity at the heart rate threshold. *Res. Q. Exerc. Sport* 64: 361–364, 1993.

3. Weir, L. L., Weir, J. P., Housh, T. J., and Johnson, G. O. Effect of an aerobic training program on physical working capacity at heart rate threshold. *Eur. J. Appl. Physiol.* 75: 351–356, 1997.

BACKGROUND

Theoretically, the physical working capacity at the ratings of perceived exertion threshold (PWC$_{RPE}$) test provides an estimate of the maximal power output that can be maintained for an extended period of time without an increase in the perception of effort during cycle ergometry.[3] The PWC$_{RPE}$ test uses the ratings of perceived exertion (RPE, 6–20) scale developed by Borg[1,2] (see figure 14.1, page 96) to assess the overall perception of effort during cycle ergometry at various submaximal power outputs. Thus, the submaximal protocol used to determine the PWC$_{RPE}$ makes it appropriate for assessing aerobic fitness in subjects where maximal exercise testing may be contraindicated, such as the elderly or clinical populations. In addition, the PWC$_{RPE}$ test is most applicable to situations where assessing the ability to perform long-term, submaximal physical activity is more important than defining a subject's maximal exercise capacity (such as maximal oxygen consumption rate, $\dot{V}O_2$max).

The PWC$_{RPE}$ test involves performing two or more eight-minute workbouts at different submaximal power outputs. This lab will describe the procedures for estimating the PWC$_{RPE}$ using two workbouts performed on the same day. Three or four workbouts, however, can also be used if the PWC$_{RPE}$ test is completed over two or more days. During each workbout, RPE values are recorded and the slope coefficient for the RPE versus time relationship is determined. The power output values are then plotted as a function of the slope coefficients for the RPE versus time relationships, and the y-intercept is defined as the PWC$_{RPE}$ (figure 14.2b). Salient features of the PWC$_{RPE}$ test are that it requires only submaximal exercise, and it can be performed using only a cycle ergometer, stopwatch, and RPE scale.

KNOW THESE TERMS & ABBREVIATIONS

☐ PWC$_{RPE}$ = physical working capacity at the ratings of perceived exertion threshold (watts), defined as the y-intercept of the power output versus RPE slope coefficient relationship (figure 14.2b)

☐ RPE = ratings of perceived exertion

☐ $\dot{V}O_2$ max = maximal oxygen consumption rate

EQUIPMENT (see Appendix 2 for vendors)	**Approximate Price**
1. Monark cycle ergometer	$2,000
2. Stopwatch	$10
3. RPE scale	$18

PROCEDURES (see photo 14.1)

The PWC$_{RPE}$ test will be performed using a Monark cycle ergometer, stopwatch, and RPE scale.

1. Prior to beginning the test: (1) adjust the seat height of the cycle ergometer to allow for near full extension of the subject's legs while pedaling, and (2) record a pre-exercise heart rate on worksheet 14.1.

2. Warm-up: The PWC$_{RPE}$ test should be preceded by a standardized warm-up protocol that includes four minutes of pedaling at 70 rpm at a resistance of 0.5 kg (power output = 34 watts).

3. The PWC$_{RPE}$ test involves two to four cycle ergometer workbouts at different power outputs.[3] Each workbout is performed at a constant pedaling cadence of 70 rpm, and the selection of power outputs for each subject usually ranges from approximately 52 (0.75 kg resistance) to 223 (3.25 kg resistance) watts.[3] See table 14.1. The power outputs should be low enough that the subject is able to complete the full eight minutes for each workbout, but high enough to elicit a positive slope in the RPE versus time relationship. For small or untrained subjects, the recommended power outputs for the PWC$_{RPE}$ test are between 52 (0.75 kg resistance) and 137 (2.0 kg resistance) watts. For large or trained subjects, as well as experienced cyclists, the recommended power outputs are between 137 (2.0 kg resistance) and 223 (3.25 kg resistance) watts. These power outputs, however, should be viewed as only recommendations. It may be necessary to adjust them up or down to ensure that the RPE versus time slope coefficient is positive and the subject is able to complete the entire eight-minute workbout.

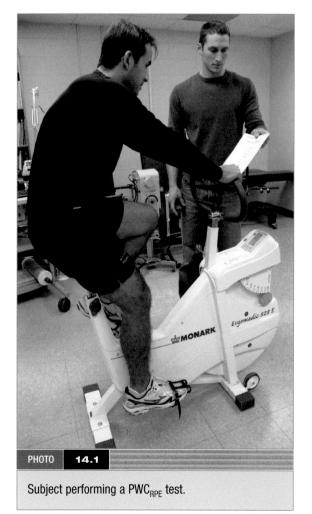

PHOTO **14.1**

Subject performing a PWC$_{RPE}$ test.

4. Following the warm-up, have the subject rest for two minutes. During this rest period, instruct the subject on how to use the RPE scale shown in figure 14.1. Provide the following instructions: "During the exercise test, we want you to pay close attention to how hard you feel the exercise work rate is. This feeling should reflect your total amount of exertion and fatigue, combining all sensations and feelings of physical stress, effort, and fatigue. Don't concern yourself with any one factor, such as leg pain, shortness of breath, or exercise intensity, but try to concentrate on your total, inner feeling of exertion. Try not to underestimate or overestimate your feelings of exertion; be as accurate as you can."

5. After the two-minute rest period, have the subject begin to pedal at 70 rpm, and set the resistance (power output) to the appropriate level as quickly as possible during the first few seconds of the workbout.

6. Once the resistance is set, begin to time the workbout with a stopwatch.

7. Give the subject verbal encouragement to maintain the 70 rpm cadence. At the end of minutes 1, 2, 3,

Resistance settings and corresponding power outputs at 70 rpm for a Monark cycle ergometer.   **TABLE   14.1**

Resistance (kg)	Power output (watts)
0.50	34
0.75	52
1.00	69
1.25	86
1.50	103
1.75	120
2.00	137
2.25	154
2.50	172
2.75	189
3.00	206
3.25	223
3.50	240
3.75	257
4.00	275

4, 5, 6, 7, and 8, show the subject the RPE scale (figure 14.1), and ask the subject for an RPE value that reflects his or her perception of effort. Record the subject's RPE value on worksheet 14.1.

8. Cool-down. After each workbout, allow the subject to continue to pedal for two to three minutes (or longer if the subject desires) with no resistance.

9. The two workbouts at different power outputs can be performed on a single day. If a second workbout is to be performed during the same laboratory visit, have the subject rest (following the cool-down) until the heart rate returns to within 10 beats per minute of the pre-exercise level to ensure that he or she is fully recovered before performing the second workbout. This usually takes at least 30 minutes.

Sample Calculations

1. Use simple linear regression analysis ($y = b(x) + a$) to calculate the slope coefficient for the RPE versus time relationship for each workbout (figure 14.2a). Simple linear regression can be performed using many handheld calculators or software (such as Microsoft Excel and others) for PC and Macintosh computers.

FIGURE	14.1	Borg rating of perceived exertion (RPE).[1,2]

INSTRUCTIONS to the Borg-RPE Scale®

During the work we want you to rate your perception of exertion, i.e., how heavy and strenuous the exercise feels to you and how tired you are. The perception of exertion is mainly felt as strain and fatigue in your muscles and as breathlessness, or aches in the chest. All work requires some effort, even if this is only minimal. This is true also if you only move a little, e.g., walking slowly.

Use this scale from 6 to 20, with 6 meaning "No exertion at all" and 20 meaning "maximal exertion."

6   "No exertion at all," means that you don't feel any exertion whatsoever, e.g., no muscle fatigue, no breathlessness or difficulties breathing.

9   "Very light" exertion, as taking a shorter walk at your own pace.

13 A "somewhat hard" work, but it still feels OK to continue.

15 It is "hard" and tiring, but continuing isn't terribly difficult.

17 "Very hard." This is very strenuous work. You can still go on, but you really have to push yourself and you are very tired.

19 An "extremely" strenuous level. For most people this is the most strenuous work they have ever experienced.

Try to appraise your feeling of exertion and fatigue as spontaneously and as honestly as possible, without thinking about what the actual physical load is. Try not to underestimate and not to overestimate your exertion. It's your own feeling of effort and exertion that is important, not how this compares with other people's. Look at the scale and the expressions and then give a number. Use any number you like on the scale, not just one of those with an explanation behind it.

Any questions?

Note: For correct usage of the scale, the exact design and instructions given in Borg's folders must be followed.

THE SCALE

6	No exertion at all
7	
8	Extremely light
9	Very light
10	
11	Light
12	
13	Somewhat hard
14	
15	Hard (heavy)
16	
17	Very hard
18	
19	Extremely hard
20	Maximal exertion

Borg RPE Scale®

©Gunnar Borg, 1970, 1985, 1998, 2004.

TIME (min)	WORKBOUT 1 RPE values	WORKBOUT 2 RPE values
1	6	8
2	6	9
3	7	10
4	8	11
5	10	11
6	11	12
7	12	14
8	13	17

For workbout 1, enter the x-values as 1, 2, 3, 4, 5, 6, 7, and 8, and the y-values as 6, 6, 7, 8, 10, 11, 12, and 13.

Workout 1 simple linear regression equation: RPE = 0.7 (time) + 4.9

Thus, for workbout 1, the RPE versus time slope coefficient = 0.7 RPE • min^{-1}.

For workout 2, enter the x-values as 1, 2, 3, 4, 5, 6, 7, and 8, and the y-values as 8, 9, 10, 11, 11, 12, 14, and 17.

Workout 2 simple linear regression equation: RPE = 1.1(time) + 6.5

Thus, for workbout 2, the RPE versus time slope coefficient = 1.1 RPE • min^{-1}.

Description of the method for estimating the physical working capacity at the ratings of perceived exertion threshold (PWC_{RPE}).   **FIGURE   14.2**

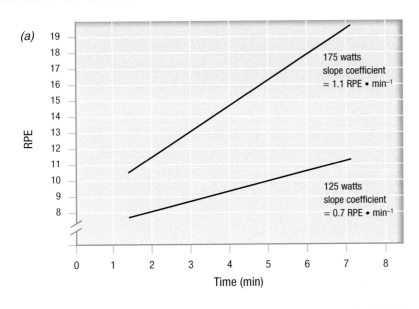

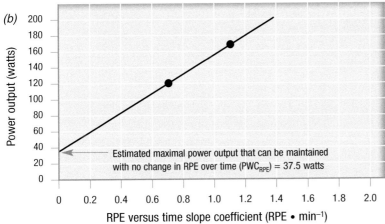

(a) The ratings of perceived exertion (RPE) data are plotted as a function of time for various power outputs on a cycle ergometer. (b) The slope coefficients from (a) are plotted for each of the power outputs, and the PWC_{RPE} is estimated as the y-intercept value.

2. Use simple linear regression analysis $(y = b(x) + a)$ to calculate the y-intercept (i.e., the PWC_{RPE}) for the power output versus RPE slope coefficient relationship (figure 14.2b).

	RPE VERSUS TIME SLOPE COEFFICIENT (RPE • min⁻¹)	POWER OUTPUT (watts)
Workbout 1	0.7	125
Workbout 2	1.1	175

Simple linear regression equation: Power output = 125 (RPE versus time slope coefficient) + 37.5.

Thus, the estimated power output that can be maintained with no change in RPE (PWC_{RPE}) = 37.5 watts.

Worksheet **14.1**	**PHYSICAL WORKING CAPACITY AT THE RATINGS OF PERCEIVED EXERTION THRESHOLD (PWC$_{RPE}$) TEST FORM**

Name _____   *Date* _____

Scat height _____

Pre-exercise heart rate _____ bpm

Power Output

Workbout 1: _____ kg of resistance × 420 [70 rpm (constant pedal cadence) × 6 meters (constant that defines the distance the flywheel travels each pedal revolution)] / 6.12 = _____ watts

Workbout 2: _____ kg of resistance × 420 / 6.12 = _____ watts

Workbout 3 (if used): _____ kg of resistance × 420 / 6.12 = _____ watts

Workbout 4 (if used): _____ kg of resistance × 420 / 6.12 = _____ watts

Time (min)	Workbout 1 RPE	Workbout 2 RPE	Workbout 3 RPE	Workbout 4 RPE
1	_____	_____	_____	_____
2	_____	_____	_____	_____
3	_____	_____	_____	_____
4	_____	_____	_____	_____
5	_____	_____	_____	_____
6	_____	_____	_____	_____
7	_____	_____	_____	_____
8	_____	_____	_____	_____

RPE versus Time Slope Coefficient

Use linear regression analysis to determine the slope coefficient for the RPE versus time relationship for each workbout: y = b(x) + a

Workbout 1: _____ RPE • min^{-1}

Workbout 2: _____ RPE • min^{-1}

Workbout 3 (if used): _____ RPE • min^{-1}

Workbout 4 (if used): _____ RPE • min^{-1}

Use linear regression analysis to determine the y-intercept (i.e., PWC$_{RPE}$) of the power output versus RPE slope coefficient relationship:

Power output = b (RPE slope coefficient) + PWC$_{RPE}$ (see figure 14.2b).

PWC$_{RPE}$ = _____ watts

EXTENSION ACTIVITIES **Worksheet 14.2**

Name *Date*

1. Two subjects performed two separate eight-minute workbouts on a cycle ergometer at the following power outputs: workbout 1 = 150 watts and workbout 2 = 200 watts. The RPE responses for each subject and workbout are shown below:

SUBJECT A

Time (min)	Workbout 1 RPE	Workbout 2 RPE
1	6	8
2	6	9
3	7	9
4	7	10
5	8	11
6	8	12
7	9	13
8	10	14

SUBJECT B

Time (min)	Workbout 1 RPE	Workbout 2 RPE
1	6	8
2	7	9
3	7	11
4	8	12
5	9	14
6	10	15
7	11	17
8	12	19

Which subject has the higher PWC_{RPE}? subject A or subject B (circle the correct choice)

2. Describe two advantages of the PWC_{RPE} test compared to a VO_2max test.

3. Use your own data to calculate your PWC_{RPE}.

EXTENSION QUESTIONS

1. What are some common mistakes that may occur in administering this lab?
2. Identify possible sources of error in this lab.
3. Assess the practicality of using this lab in the field.
4. Research the reliability and/or validity of this lab using the Internet, journal articles, and other credible sources.

REFERENCES

1. Borg, G. Perceived exertion as an indicator of somatic stress. *Scand. J. Rehabil. Med.* 2: 92–98, 1970.
2. Borg, G. *Borg's perceived exertion and pain scales.* Champaign, IL: Human Kinetics, 1998.
3. Mielke, M., Housh, T. J., Malek, M. H., Beck, T. W., Schmidt, R. J., and Johnson, G. O. Rating of perceived exertion based tests of physical working capacity. *J. Strength Cond. Res.* 22: 293–302, 2008.

MUSCULAR STRENGTH

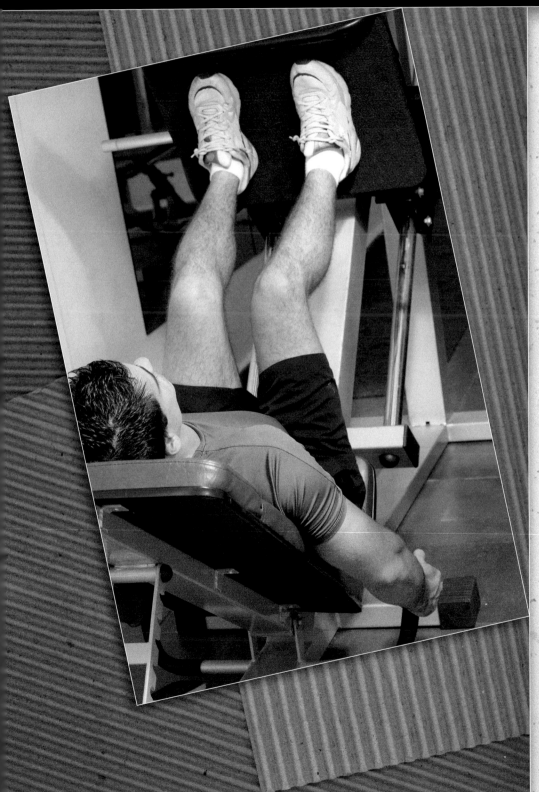

Lab 15

Assessment of Isometric
Hand Grip Strength

Lab 16

Determination of
One-Repetition Maximum
Bench Press and Leg
Press Strength

BACKGROUND

Isometric hand grip strength is an important component of physical fitness and provides a simple method for characterizing overall body strength.[1,2] The performance of many manual labor activities, such as yard and garden work and lifting and carrying large objects, depends on a certain degree of hand grip strength. Thus, the purpose of this lab is to describe the procedures for measuring isometric hand grip strength with a hand grip dynamometer.

KNOW THESE TERMS & ABBREVIATIONS

- ☐ hand grip dynamometer = an instrument that measures isometric hand grip strength, which provides a simple method for characterizing overall body strength

- ☐ isometric strength = tension production by a muscle without movement at the joint or shortening of the muscle fibers

- ☐ percentile rank = in this lab, a score between 10% and 90% that shows how the subject performed relative to others in the age group. A percentile ranking of 70, for example, indicates that the subject's grip strength is higher than 70% of the others in the age group and lower than 30% of the others in the age group.

EQUIPMENT (see Appendix 2 for vendors)   Approximate Price

Hand grip dynamometer $300

PROCEDURES

The isometric hand grip strength test can be performed using a variety of dynamometers (photo 15.1).

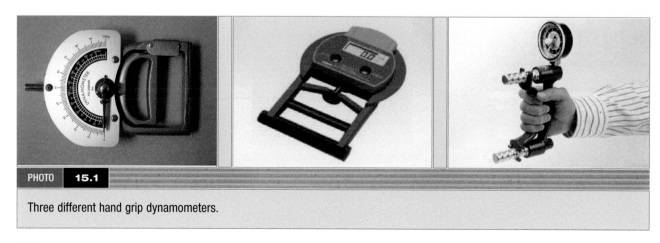

PHOTO 15.1

Three different hand grip dynamometers.

1. Prior to beginning the test, adjust the length of the handle on the hand grip dynamometer such that it feels comfortable in the hand. For individuals with very small hands, the handle of the dynamometer should be shortened, while for those with very large hands, the handle should be lengthened.[1]

2. Have the subject hold the hand grip dynamometer in the right hand with the palm facing up and the elbow at approximately 90 degrees (photo 15.2). When ready, the subject should squeeze the dynamometer maximally for three seconds. Read the force value (kg) from the dynamometer and record it on worksheet 15.1. Perform the strength test two more times with the right hand, separating the trials by two minutes of rest.

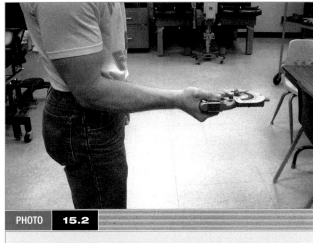

PHOTO **15.2**

The correct elbow position for performing the hand grip dynamometer strength test.

3. Repeat the procedures described in step 2 for the left hand.

4. Add the highest strength value (kg) for the right hand to that from the left hand and record the value on worksheet 15.1. Divide the sum by body weight in kg and record this value on worksheet 15.1.

5. Percentile rank norms by age and gender are provided in tables 15.1 through 15.4. Compare the sum of right and left hand grip strength to the values in tables 15.1 and 15.2 based on age and gender. Compare the sum of right and left hand grip strength divided by body weight to the values in tables 15.3 and 15.4 based on age and gender.

Percentile ranks for sum of grip strengths (kg, right plus left) for males.   TABLE   15.1

Percentile rank	Age (yrs)																
	10	11	12	13	14	15	16	17	18	19	20–24	25–29	30–34	35–39	40–44	45–49	50–59
90	34	42	52	69	89	96	106	111	117	118	122	123	124	123	123	116	110
80	30	37	47	60	80	90	99	105	106	113	115	115	115	115	115	108	102
70	26	34	41	53	72	84	95	99	101	109	110	110	110	109	108	104	96
60	24	32	38	48	66	80	91	93	98	104	105	107	106	106	103	99	93
50	22	29	34	44	61	76	87	89	96	101	102	103	102	102	100	95	89
40	20	26	31	42	58	73	84	85	93	98	99	100	98	98	97	91	85
30	18	23	30	39	54	69	78	81	90	94	94	95	95	93	93	82	81
20	15	21	27	34	49	64	74	76	86	90	89	90	90	88	87	81	75
10	11	16	23	28	39	55	68	70	81	84	80	81	82	79	81	75	66

Adapted from Montoye, H. J., and Lamphiear, D. E. Grip and arm strength in males and females, age 10 to 69. *Research Quarterly for Exercise and Sport*, Vol. 48, pp. 109–120, 1977. Reprinted with permission.

TABLE	15.2	Percentile ranks for sum of grip strengths (kg, right plus left) for females.

Percentile rank	Age (yrs)																
	10	11	12	13	14	15	16	17	18	19	20–24	25–29	30–34	35–39	40–44	45–49	50–59
90	30	37	44	49	65	60	58	61	59	63	61	67	65	66	64	64	57
80	25	33	40	44	50	54	53	54	55	59	57	62	60	59	58	57	52
70	22	30	36	41	48	49	49	50	52	54	53	57	57	55	54	53	48
60	20	27	33	38	44	45	48	47	49	50	50	53	53	53	51	52	45
50	18	25	31	36	41	43	43	44	46	48	48	49	49	51	49	49	43
40	17	23	28	34	39	41	41	42	43	46	45	48	47	49	47	47	40
30	15	20	26	32	36	38	39	39	39	42	42	46	44	46	43	44	38
20	14	17	22	30	32	36	36	36	36	39	38	43	41	43	40	40	34
10	10	12	18	26	27	31	33	31	31	36	34	37	36	36	36	34	30

Adapted from Montoye, H. J., and Lamphiear, D. E. Grip and arm strength in males and females, age 10 to 69. *Research Quarterly for Exercise and Sport,* Vol. 48, pp. 109–120, 1977. Reprinted with permission.

TABLE	15.3	Percentile ranks for ratio of sum of grip strengths to body weight (kg/kg body weight) for males.

Percentile rank	Age (yrs)																
	10	11	12	13	14	15	16	17	18	19	20–24	25–29	30–34	35–39	40–49	50–59
90	0.89	1.04	1.10	1.20	1.40	1.45	1.56	1.62	1.62	1.75	1.73	1.72	1.64	1.62	1.54	1.39
80	0.83	0.94	0.97	1.13	1.28	1.36	1.49	1.48	1.50	1.54	1.59	1.54	1.52	1.51	1.41	1.30
70	0.76	0.85	0.93	1.03	1.23	1.29	1.43	1.44	1.47	1.44	1.53	1.47	1.45	1.42	1.34	1.22
60	0.69	0.80	0.86	0.98	1.15	1.25	1.39	1.39	1.44	1.36	1.45	1.40	1.39	1.35	1.28	1.19
50	0.65	0.77	0.80	0.93	1.09	1.22	1.30	1.35	1.37	1.33	1.39	1.35	1.33	1.28	1.24	1.14
40	0.62	0.71	0.74	0.86	1.02	1.17	1.19	1.28	1.33	1.29	1.32	1.28	1.29	1.23	1.19	1.10
30	0.52	0.66	0.70	0.80	0.96	1.14	1.14	1.21	1.31	1.24	1.26	1.20	1.24	1.17	1.14	1.03
20	0.45	0.58	0.66	0.77	0.90	1.06	1.09	1.16	1.22	1.17	1.18	1.12	1.18	1.11	1.07	0.98
10	0.38	0.48	0.61	0.65	0.81	0.95	0.98	1.01	1.16	1.12	1.08	1.01	1.10	1.02	0.99	0.89

Adapted from Montoye, H. J., and Lamphiear, D. E. Grip and arm strength in males and females, age 10 to 69. *Research Quarterly for Exercise and Sport,* Vol. 48, pp. 109–120, 1977. Reprinted with permission.

Percentile rank	Age (yrs)															
	10	11	12	13	14	15	16	17	18	19	20–24	25–29	30–34	35–39	40–49	50–59
90	0.71	0.91	0.92	0.96	1.08	1.04	0.98	1.12	1.02	1.10	1.04	1.12	1.05	1.07	1.02	0.90
80	0.65	0.80	0.80	0.86	0.96	0.92	0.94	1.02	0.95	1.04	0.97	1.02	1.00	1.00	0.93	0.83
70	0.62	0.72	0.75	0.81	0.86	0.89	0.84	0.96	0.90	0.94	0.91	0.97	0.94	0.93	0.87	0.78
60	0.57	0.68	0.72	0.79	0.81	0.84	0.79	0.89	0.82	0.85	0.86	0.91	0.89	0.87	0.81	0.71
50	0.54	0.64	0.66	0.73	0.76	0.79	0.76	0.83	0.78	0.80	0.81	0.86	0.83	0.84	0.77	0.68
40	0.50	0.57	0.61	0.68	0.71	0.76	0.73	0.78	0.72	0.77	0.77	0.82	0.78	0.80	0.73	0.63
30	0.46	0.53	0.57	0.65	0.67	0.69	0.71	0.71	0.69	0.74	0.72	0.75	0.72	0.75	0.69	0.59
20	0.42	0.45	0.54	0.63	0.65	0.65	0.65	0.66	0.65	0.69	0.68	0.68	0.66	0.69	0.63	0.52
10	0.32	0.33	0.47	0.52	0.58	0.57	0.57	0.52	0.58	0.64	0.61	0.61	0.60	0.60	0.54	0.48

Percentile ranks for ratio of sum of grip strengths to body weight (kg/kg body weight) for females. — TABLE 15.4

Adapted from Montoye, H. J., and Lamphiear, D. E. Grip and arm strength in males and females, age 10 to 69. *Research Quarterly for Exercise and Sport,* Vol. 48, pp. 109–120, 1977. Reprinted with permission.

Sample Calculations

Name: _I. M. Strong_

Gender: _Male_

Age: _21 years_

Body weight: _75 kg_

	Trial 1 (kg)	Trial 2 (kg)	Trial 3 (kg)	Max of three trials (kg)
Right hand	50	52	53	53
Left hand	51	50	52	52

Sum of right and left = _105_ kg

Approximate percentile rank = _60_ (table 15.1)

Sum of right and left (kg)	Body weight (kg)	Grip strength ratio (kg/kg body weight)
105	75	1.40

Sum of right and left (kg) _105_ / Body weight (kg) _75_ = Grip strength ratio (kg/kg body weight) _1.40_

Approximate percentile rank = _51_ (table 15.3)

Worksheet 15.1	ISOMETRIC HAND GRIP STRENGTH FORM

Name _____   Date _____

Age: _____   Gender: _____

	Trial 1 (kg)	Trial 2 (kg)	Trial 3 (kg)	Max of three trials (kg)
Right hand	54	~~53~~	57	57
Left hand	53	54	59	59

Sum of right plus left ____116____

Percentile rank (see tables 15.1 and 15.2) = ____80____

Sum of right and left (kg)	Body weight (kg)	Grip strength ratio (kg/kg body weight)
116	/ 66	= 1.7

Percentile rank (see tables 15.3 and 15.4): ____90____

Worksheet 15.2	EXTENSION ACTIVITIES

Name _____   Date _____

1. Using your own data, report the sum of your right and left hand grip strength scores (kg) and percentile ranking.

   116

2. Using your own data, report the ratio of the sum of your grip strengths to body weight (kg/kg body weight) and percentile ranking.

3. Describe three activities that you regularly perform that depend on possessing a high degree of hand grip strength.

   finger tip push ups, Catching football, Grabbing Back Packs opening car door

4. Describe three sporting activities that, in part, require a high degree of hand grip strength.

   football, wrestling, Basketball

EXTENSION QUESTIONS

1. What are some common mistakes that may occur in administering this lab?

2. Identify possible sources of error in this lab.

3. Assess the practicality of using this lab in the field.

4. Research the reliability and/or validity of this lab using the Internet, journal articles, and other credible sources.

REFERENCES

1. Montoye, H. J., and Faulkner, J. A. Determination of the optimum setting of an adjustable grip dynamometer. *Res. Q.* 35: 29–36, 1964.

2. Montoye, H. J., and Lamphiear, D. E. Grip and arm strength in males and females, age 10 to 69. *Res. Q.* 48: 109–120, 1977.

Lab 16 — Determination of One-Repetition Maximum Bench Press and Leg Press Strength

BACKGROUND

The one-repetition maximum, or 1-RM, refers to the maximum amount of weight that can be lifted one time. The 1-RM is a standard index to quantify muscle strength. A 1-RM determination can be made for any dynamic constant external resistance (DCER; formerly known as isotonic) strength exercise, such as the bench press, leg extension and flexion, leg press, squat, or power clean. In addition, 1-RM testing can be performed using free weights or machine exercises. The procedure is a trial-and-error method where, after a warm-up period, progressively heavier weights are lifted one time until the subject cannot successfully complete the lift of a given weight.[1] The weight is then reduced until the heaviest successful weight is determined.

In performing 1-RM testing for a given exercise it is helpful (but not required) to have subjects with some minimal level of weightlifting experience, because strength exercises are a motor skill that improves with practice. Therefore, a 1-RM value is affected not only by the subject's strength, but also by the subject's skill in performing the task. In addition, prior experience allows subjects to estimate their strength more accurately prior to testing. This estimate helps eliminate unnecessary lifts that are either too easy or too hard, so that the testing is efficient and the effects of fatigue are minimized.

In this laboratory you will learn to perform 1-RM strength testing for bench press and leg press exercises. You will also compare the 1-RM strength values to age- and gender-specific norms. Percentile rank norms for strength relative to body weight (1-RM strength in lbs/body weight in lbs) are provided in tables 16.1 through 16.4 for the bench press and leg press exercises for males and females.

Bench Press

The bench press is a common exercise in both training and testing (see photos 16.1 and 16.2). The motion of the bench press is analogous to a push-up, except the subject lies on his or her back and the resistance is supplied by a barbell or a bench press machine. The pectoral muscles, triceps brachii, and anterior deltoid muscles are the primary muscles

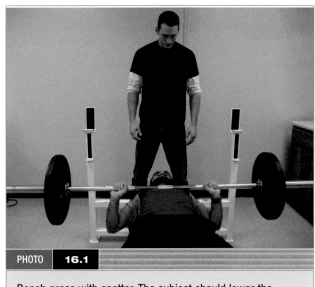

PHOTO 16.1

Bench press with spotter. The subject should lower the weight slowly until the barbell touches the mid-chest.

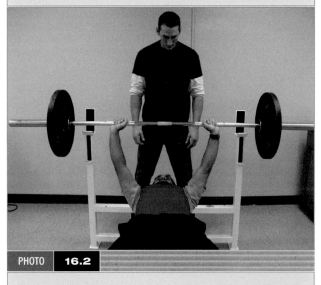

PHOTO 16.2

Bench press with spotter. During ascent and descent the forearms should be vertical to the floor and parallel to each other.

involved in the lift. Because the use of a barbell requires that the subject balance the resistance in addition to lifting the weight, the 1-RM from a free weight bench press may be quite different from the 1-RM determined on a machine. Further, because the mechanics of the different machines vary, the 1-RM from the same subject on different machines may also differ substantially. These factors should be kept in mind when interpreting the results relative to the normative values provided in tables 16.1 and 16.2.

Percentile rank norms for bench press 1-RM relative to body weight by age for males.[3] **TABLE 16.1**

Percentile rank	20–29	30–39	40–49	50–59	60–69
90	1.48	1.24	1.10	0.97	0.89
80	1.32	1.12	1.00	0.90	0.82
70	1.22	1.04	0.93	0.84	0.77
60	1.14	0.98	0.88	0.79	0.72
50	1.06	0.93	0.84	0.75	0.68
40	0.99	0.88	0.80	0.71	0.66
30	0.93	0.83	0.76	0.68	0.63
20	0.88	0.78	0.72	0.63	0.57
10	0.80	0.71	0.65	0.57	0.53

Note: Values are bench press 1-RM in lbs/body weight in lbs.

Percentile rank norms for bench press 1-RM relative to body weight by age for females.[3] **TABLE 16.2**

Percentile rank	20–29	30–39	40–49	50–59	60–69
90	0.54	0.49	0.46	0.40	0.41
80	0.49	0.45	0.40	0.37	0.38
70	0.42	0.42	0.38	0.35	0.36
60	0.41	0.41	0.37	0.33	0.32
50	0.40	0.38	0.34	0.31	0.30
40	0.37	0.37	0.32	0.28	0.29
30	0.35	0.34	0.30	0.26	0.28
20	0.33	0.32	0.27	0.23	0.26
10	0.30	0.27	0.23	0.19	0.25

Note: Values are bench press 1-RM in lbs/body weight in lbs.

When using free weights, a failed attempt to lift a weight may result in injury if the bar becomes out of control. Therefore, an experienced "spotter" should be ready to help the subject lift the weight when the attempt is clearly going to fail.[2] Most bench press machines do not require the use of a spotter.

For the free weight bench press, the subject should lie supine on the bench with both feet flat on the floor with the buttocks and shoulders in contact with the bench. The subject should grip the barbell with a closed grip. That is, the thumb should wrap around the barbell so that it cannot roll out of the hand. Grip width should be slightly wider than the shoulders and evenly spaced so that the load is the same on each arm. The barbell should then be removed from the bench press racks. The spotter may help the subject by assisting the "liftoff." After the liftoff, the subject should lower the weight slowly until the barbell touches the mid-chest.[2] This should take one to two seconds. As soon as the barbell touches the chest, the subject should lift it upward until the elbows are locked. During the descent and ascent, the forearms should be parallel to each other and oriented vertical to the floor.[2] After the lift, the spotter may help the subject place the barbell on the racks. Lifts are not acceptable if the barbell bounces off the chest or if the buttocks come off the bench.

Leg Press (see photos 16.3 and 16.4)

The leg press is a machine-based exercise that primarily involves the simultaneous activation of the leg extensors (quadriceps) and hip extensors (gluteal muscles and hamstrings). There are several different types of machines, and the body position can vary considerably from machine to machine, which will affect the amount of weight that can be lifted. Therefore, as with the bench press, caution should be used when interpreting the normative leg press values in tables 16.3 and 16.4. Most machines allow you to alter the angle between the torso and thigh, and, if possible, this should be set to about 90 degrees.[2]

At the start of the lift, the feet should be about shoulder-width apart and the toes pointed up or in a slightly "toe out" position. The shoulders and buttocks should be firmly braced against the machine.[2] Most leg press machines have hand grips that the subject can use to help stabilize the torso during the

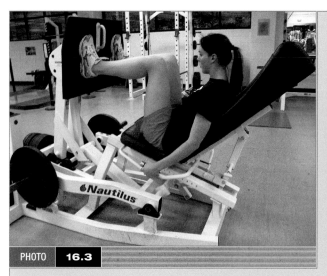

PHOTO **16.3**

Leg press. The subject lowers the weight slowly until the angle at the knee reaches approximately 90 degrees.

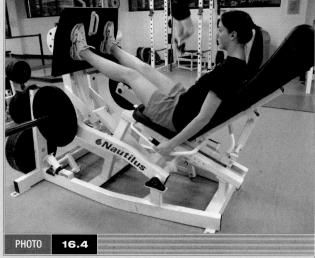

PHOTO **16.4**

Leg press. The subject should keep the legs in line with the hips and ankles.

lift. Once positioned, the subject will unrack the weight so that the legs are fully extended (although the legs should not be hyperextended at the start of the lift). From full extension, the subject lowers the weight slowly until the angle at the knee joint reaches approximately 90 degrees (photo 16.3), and then extends the legs and hips until the legs are again fully extended (photo 16.4). The subject should keep the legs in line with the hips and ankles, so that the legs do not track in (knock-kneed) or out.[2]

Percentile rank norms for leg press 1-RM relative to body weight by age for males.[3]   **TABLE   16.3**

Percentile rank	20–29	30–39	40–49	50–59	60–69
90	2.27	2.07	1.92	1.80	1.73
80	2.13	1.93	1.82	1.71	1.62
70	2.05	1.85	1.74	1.64	1.56
60	1.97	1.77	1.68	1.58	1.49
50	1.91	1.71	1.62	1.52	1.43
40	1.83	1.65	1.57	1.46	1.38
30	1.74	1.59	1.51	1.39	1.30
20	1.63	1.52	1.44	1.32	1.25
10	1.51	1.43	1.35	1.22	1.16

Note: Values are leg press 1-RM in lbs/body weight in lbs.

Percentile rank norms for leg press 1-RM relative to body weight by age for females.[3]   **TABLE   16.4**

Percentile rank	20–29	30–39	40–49	50–59	60–69
90	2.05	1.73	1.63	1.51	1.40
80	1.66	1.50	1.46	1.30	1.25
70	1.42	1.47	1.35	1.24	1.18
60	1.36	1.32	1.26	1.18	1.15
50	1.32	1.26	1.19	1.09	1.08
40	1.25	1.21	1.12	1.03	1.04
30	1.23	1.16	1.03	0.95	0.98
20	1.13	1.09	0.94	0.86	0.94
10	1.02	0.94	0.76	0.75	0.84

Note: Values are leg press 1-RM in lbs/body weight in lbs.

KNOW THESE TERMS & ABBREVIATIONS

☐ DCER = dynamic constant external resistance

☐ 1-RM = one-repetition maximum, a standard index to quantify muscle strength that refers to the maximum amount of weight that can be lifted one time

☐ leg extensors = the quadriceps, made up of the rectus femoris, vastus lateralis, vastus intermedius, and vastus medialis

☐ hip extensors = the gluteal muscles (gluteus maximus and gluteus medius) and the hamstrings (biceps femoris, semitendinosus, and semimembranosus)

☐ hyperextension = extension of a joint beyond the normal range of motion

EQUIPMENT (see Appendix 2 for vendors)	**Approximate Price**
1. Standard Olympic weight plates	$0.69/lb
2. Olympic bar	$150
3. Bench press rack	$300–$500
4. Leg press machine	$1,400–$1,600
5. Stopwatch	$10

PROCEDURES (see photos 16.1 to 16.4)

1. Have the subject estimate his or her 1-RM strength and record it on worksheet 16.1.

2. Have the subject perform a general warm-up (three to five minutes) of the body area to be tested.

3. Continue the warm-up by performing eight repetitions at a weight equal to 50% of the estimated 1-RM and three repetitions at 70% of the estimated 1-RM.

4. To determine the 1-RM, perform a single repetition at a heavier weight than that used during the warm-up. The increase in weight should be based on the relative ease or difficulty of the set in the warm-up.

5. Repeat performing single repetitions using progressively heavier weights until a weight is reached that cannot be successfully lifted. Adjust the increases in weight so that increments are approximately evenly spaced and so that at least two single lifts are performed between the weight used in the warm-up and the estimated 1-RM.

6. At failure, decrease the weight to a level approximately midway between the last successful lift and the weight at failure.

7. Repeat using heavier or lighter weights until the desired level of precision is achieved (usually within about 5 lbs) and record the 1-RM weight on worksheet 16.1.

8. Rest intervals between single lifts should be between one and five minutes.[4,5]

9. Try to determine the 1-RM in about three to five single lifts, excluding warm-up lifts.[1]

10. To increase time efficiency, more than one subject can be tested at a given station, so that one person is performing lifts while the others are resting.

Sample Calculations

Name: _I. M. Strong_

Gender: _male_

Body weight: _180 lbs_

Age: _21 years_

Mode of lift: _Bench press_

Estimated 1-RM: _200 lbs_

WARM-UP

1. _8_ repetitions at _100_ lbs (approximately 50% of estimated 1-RM)

2. _3_ repetitions at _140_ lbs (approximately 70% of estimated 1-RM)

1-RM TESTING

1. *Circle:* (success) failure at _170_ lbs

2. *Circle:* (success) failure at _185_ lbs

3. *Circle:* success (failure) at _200_ lbs

4. *Circle:* (success) failure at _195_ lbs

5. *Circle:* success failure at _____ lbs

6. *Circle:* success failure at _____ lbs

7. *Circle:* success failure at _____ lbs

1-RM/body weight: _195 lbs/180 lbs_ = _1.08_

Percentile rank classification for 1-RM in lbs/body weight in lbs

= _52nd percentile_ (see tables 16.1–16.4)

Worksheet 16.1   DETERMINATION OF ONE-REPETITION MAXIMUM STRENGTH

Name _____   *Date* _____

Gender: _____

Body Weight: _____ lbs

Age: _____

Mode of lift: _____

Estimated 1-RM lbs: _____

WARM-UP

1. _____ repetitions at _____ lbs (approximately 50% of estimated 1-RM)

2. _____ repetitions at _____ lbs (approximately 70% of estimated 1-RM)

1-RM TESTING

1. *Circle:*   success   failure   at _____ lbs

2. *Circle:*   success   failure   at _____ lbs

3. *Circle:*   success   failure   at _____ lbs

4. *Circle:*   success   failure   at _____ lbs

5. *Circle:*   success   failure   at _____ lbs

6. *Circle:*   success   failure   at _____ lbs

7. *Circle:*   success   failure   at _____ lbs

1-RM/body weight _____

Percentile rank classification for 1-RM in lbs/body weight in lbs = _____ (see tables 16.1–16.4)

Name _____   Date _____

1. Given the following data, answer the questions below.

   Gender: _____*female*_____

   Age: ___*22 years*___

   Bench press 1-RM: _____*70 lbs*_____

   Body weight: ____*150 lbs*____

   Bench press 1-RM in lbs./body weight in lbs: _____

   Percentile rank = _____ (see table 16.2)

2. Given the following data, answer the questions below.

   Gender: _____*male*_____

   Age: ___*44 years*___

   Leg press 1-RM: ____*275 lbs*____

   Body weight: ____*180 lbs*____

   Leg press 1-RM in lbs/body weight in lbs: _____

   Percentile rank = _____ (see table 16.3)

EXTENSION QUESTIONS

1. What are some common mistakes that may occur in administering this lab?

2. Identify possible sources of error in this lab.

3. Assess the practicality of using this lab in the field.

4. Research the reliability and/or validity of this lab using the Internet, journal articles, and other credible sources.

REFERENCES

1. Brown, L. E., and Weir, J. P. ASEP Procedures Recommendation I: Accurate assessment of muscular strength and power. *J. Exercise Phys. Online* 4: 1–21, 2001.

2. Graham, J. F. Resistance exercise techniques and spotting. In *Conditioning for Strength and Human Performance*, eds. T. J. Chandler and L. E. Brown. Baltimore: Lippincott Williams & Wilkins, 2008, pp. 182–236.

3. Hoffman, J. *Norms for Fitness, Performance, and Health*. Champaign, IL: Human Kinetics, 2006.

4. Matuszak, M. E., Fry, A. C., Weiss, L. W., Ireland, T. R., and McNight, M. M. Effect of rest interval length on repeated 1 repetition maximum back squats. *J. Strength Cond. Res.* 17: 634–637, 2003.

5. Weir, J. P., Wagner, L. L., and Housh, T. J. The effect of rest interval length on repeated maximal bench presses. *J. Strength Cond. Res.* 8: 58–60, 1994.

Unit 5

MUSCULAR ENDURANCE

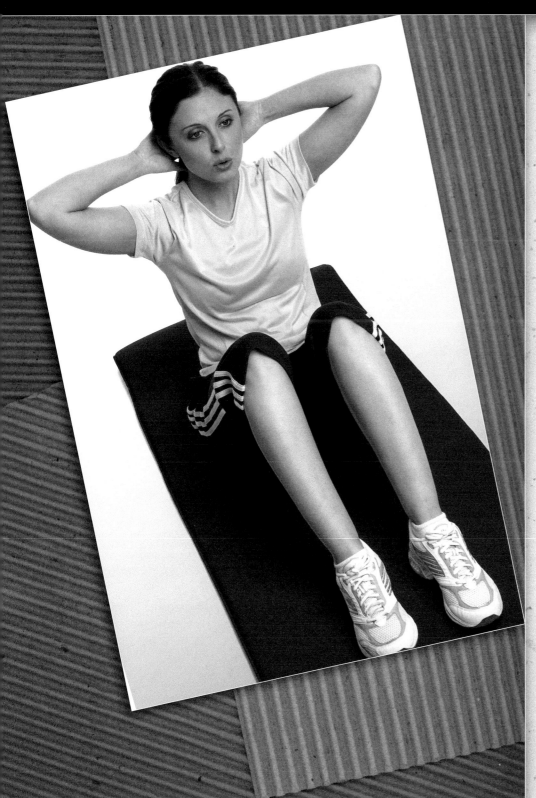

Lab 17
1-Minute Sit-up Test
of Muscular Endurance

Lab 18
Push-up Test of Upper-Body
Muscular Endurance

1-Minute Sit-up Test of Muscular Endurance

BACKGROUND

Muscular endurance describes the ability to perform repeated muscle actions.[1,2,3,4] Muscular endurance is an important component of physical fitness, because most activities of daily living as well as sporting activities require multiple submaximal muscle actions. For example, household activities such as gardening, lawn mowing, shoveling snow, and vacuuming require repeated actions that often utilize the same muscles. Furthermore, although success in some sports, such as power lifting and Olympic lifting, is based on the ability to perform a single, maximal muscle action, most sports, such as rowing, swimming, cross-country skiing, bicycling, wrestling, boxing, sprinting, baseball pitching, and many others, involve repeated muscle actions. Thus, although muscular strength and muscular endurance are typically related, they involve the assessment of separate components of physical fitness.

The 1-Minute Sit-up Test is commonly used to assess the endurance of the abdominal muscles. Poor abdominal muscle endurance (as well as strength) is often thought to contribute to low back pain.[1] Thus, the 1-Minute Sit-up Test can provide valuable information about the potential risk of developing low back pain.

In this laboratory, you will learn to conduct the 1-Minute Sit-up Test of muscular endurance and to compare the results of the test to the norms in tables 17.1 and 17.2 to classify the subject based on age and gender.[3]

KNOW THESE TERMS & ABBREVIATIONS

☐ muscular endurance = the ability to perform repeated muscle actions that often utilize the same muscles

TABLE 17.1 Male norms for the 1-Minute Sit-Up Test (number of correctly performed sit-ups).[3,4]

Classification	Age (years)					
	18–25	26–35	36–45	46–55	56–65	66+
Excellent	60–50	55–46	50–42	50–36	42–32	40–29
Good	48–45	45–41	40–36	33–29	29–26	26–22
Above average	42–40	38–36	34–30	28–25	24–21	21–20
Average	38–36	34–32	29–28	24–22	20–17	18–16
Below average	34–32	30–29	26–24	21–18	16–13	14–12
Poor	30–26	28–24	22–18	17–13	12–9	10–8
Very poor	24–12	21–6	16–4	12–4	8–2	6–2

Female norms for the 1-Minute Sit-Up Test (number of correctly performed sit-ups).[3,4] **TABLE 17.2**

Classification	Age (years)					
	18–25	26–35	36–45	46–55	56–65	66+
Excellent	55–44	54–40	50–34	42–28	38–25	36–24
Good	41–37	37–33	30–27	25–22	21–18	22–18
Above average	36–33	32–29	26–24	21–18	17–13	16–14
Average	32–29	28–25	22–20	17–14	12–10	13–11
Below average	28–25	24–21	18–16	13–10	9–7	10–6
Poor	24–20	20–16	14–10	9–6	6–4	4–2
Very poor	17–4	12–1	6–1	4–0	2–0	1–0

☐ muscular strength = the maximal force that can be exerted by a specific muscle or muscle group

EQUIPMENT
(see Appendix 2 for vendors)

Approximate Price

Floor mat $20

PROCEDURES[3,4]

1. Have the subject lie on his or her back, with knees bent, feet flat on the floor, and fingers next to the ears. The subject's heels should be approximately 18 inches from the buttocks (photo 17.1). Have a partner hold the subject's feet firmly on the floor for stability.[3,4]

2. The subject should touch each elbow to the opposite knee, alternately, and perform as many sit-ups as possible in one minute (photo 17.2). The partner should count the number of sit-ups correctly performed during the test.[3,4]

3. Record the number of correctly performed sit-ups on worksheet 17.1.

Sample Classification

Gender: _Female_

Age: _37 years_

Number of sit-ups in one minute: _36_

Classification (see table 17.2): _excellent_

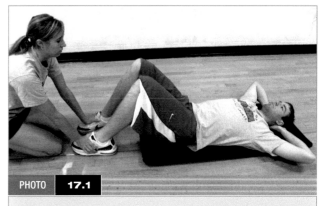

PHOTO **17.1**

Sit-up test. The subject's heels should be approximately 18 inches from the buttocks.

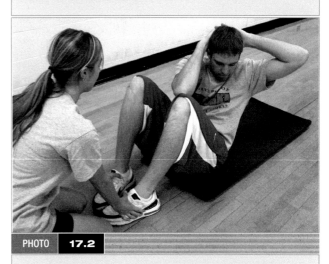

PHOTO **17.2**

Sit-up test. A partner holds the subject's feet firmly on the floor while the subject touches each elbow to the opposite knee.

| Worksheet **17.1** | THE 1-MINUTE SIT-UP TEST FORM |

Name _____   Date _____

Gender: _____Male_____

Age: _____22_____

1. Number of correctly performed sit-ups = _____43_____

2. Classification = ___Above Average_____ (see tables 17.1 and 17.2)

| Worksheet **17.2** | EXTENSION ACTIVITIES |

Name _____   Date _____

1. Given the following data, classify the results of a 1-Minute Sit-up Test.

   Gender: _____female_____

   Age: _____26 years_____

   Number of sit-ups in 1 minute: _____29_____

   Classification = ___Above Average___ (see table 17.2).

2. Given the following data, classify the results of a 1-Minute Sit-up Test.

   Gender: _____male_____

   Age: _____20 years_____

   Number of sit-ups in 1 minute: _____33_____

   Classification = ___below Average___ (see table 17.1).

EXTENSION QUESTIONS

1. What are some common mistakes that may occur in administering this lab?

2. Identify possible sources of error in this lab.

3. Assess the practicality of using this lab in the field.

4. Research the reliability and/or validity of this lab using the Internet, journal articles, and other credible sources.

REFERENCES

1. American College of Sports Medicine. *ACSM's Guidelines for Exercise Testing and Prescription*, 7th edition. Philadelphia: Lippincott Williams & Wilkins, 2006, pp. 83–85.

2. Cramer, J. T., and Coburn, J. W. Fitness testing protocols and norms. In *NSCA's Essentials of Personal Training*, eds. R. W. Earle and T. K. Baechle. Champaign, IL: Human Kinetics, 2004.

3. Golding, L. A., Myers, C. R., and Sinning, W. E. *Y's Way to Physical Fitness*, 3rd edition. Champaign, IL: Human Kinetics, 1989, pp. 111–124.

4. Morrow, J. R., Jackson, A. W., Disch, J. G., and Mood, D. P. *Measurement of Evaluation in Human Performance*, 3rd edition. Champaign, IL: Human Kinetics, 2005, pp. 251–252.

Lab 18

Push-up Test of Upper-Body Muscular Endurance

BACKGROUND

Muscular endurance, an important component of physical fitness, describes the ability to perform repeated muscle actions.[1,2,3] Muscular endurance contributes to our ability to accomplish many activities of daily living, such as gardening, lawn mowing, and shoveling snow. In addition, a number of sports, such as rowing, swimming, wrestling, and many others, require substantial muscular endurance to compete successfully.

The ability to perform repeated muscle actions is specific to the muscle group involved.[3] For example, depending on training status and/or the competitive sport, an individual may demonstrate considerable upper-body muscular endurance, but display less lower-body or abdominal muscular endurance. Thus, testing procedures are often designed to assess upper-body, lower-body, or abdominal muscular endurance.[1,2,3]

In this laboratory, you will learn to administer the Push-up Test of Upper-Body Muscular Endurance and to classify the subject based on age and gender.[1]

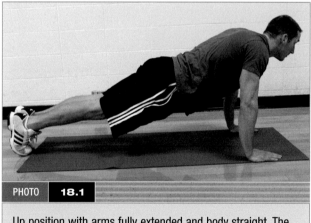

PHOTO **18.1**

Up position with arms fully extended and body straight. The hands should be pointed forward and approximately shoulder-width apart. Male subjects use the toes as the pivot point.

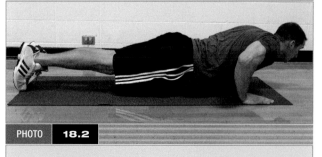

PHOTO **18.2**

The subject lowers the body until the chin touches the floor.

KNOW THESE TERMS & ABBREVIATIONS

☐ muscular endurance = the ability to perform repeated muscle actions that often utilize the same muscles

EQUIPMENT
(see Appendix 2 for vendors)

	Approximate Price
Floor mat	$20

PROCEDURES[1,3] (see photos 18.1 to 18.4)

1. Have the subject begin in the up position with arms fully extended and body straight. The hands should be pointed forward and approximately shoulder-width apart (see photos 18.1 and 18.3). Male subjects use the toes as the pivot point. Female subjects should assume the "modified knee push-up" position with the knees bent and touching the floor (see photo 18.3).

2. The subject lowers his or her body until the chin touches the floor (see photos 18.2 and 18.4) and then returns to the up position by straightening the elbows.

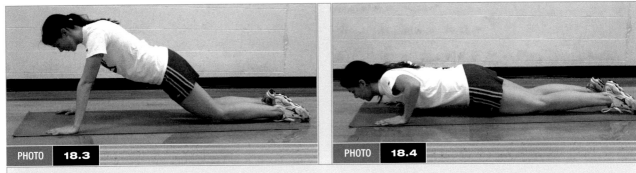

PHOTO **18.3**

Up position with arms fully extended and body straight. The hands should be pointed forward and approximately shoulder-width apart. Female subjects should assume the "modified knee push-up" position with the knees bent and touching the floor.

PHOTO **18.4**

The subject lowers the body until the chin touches the floor.

3. A partner should count the number of push-ups performed correctly to exhaustion without stopping.
4. Record the number of correctly performed push-ups on worksheet 18.1.

Sample Classification

Gender: _Male_

Age: _23 years_

Number of consecutive push-ups to exhaustion: _28_

Classification (see table 18.1): _good_

Norms for the push-up test of upper body muscular endurance.[3]   TABLE   **18.1**

Category	Age (years)									
	20–29		30–39		40–49		50–59		60–69	
GENDER	MALE	FEMALE	MALE	FEMALE	MALE	FEMALE	MALE	FEMALE	MALE	FEMALE
Excellent	36	30	30	27	25	24	21	21	18	17
Very good	35	29	29	26	24	23	20	20	17	16
	29	21	22	20	17	15	13	11	11	12
Good	28	20	21	19	16	14	12	10	10	11
	22	15	17	13	13	11	10	7	8	5
Fair	21	14	16	12	12	10	9	6	7	4
	17	10	12	8	10	5	7	2	5	2
Needs improvement	16	9	11	7	9	4	6	1	4	1

| Worksheet **18.1** | PUSH-UP TEST OF UPPER-BODY MUSCULAR ENDURANCE FORM |

Name _____   Date _____

Gender: _____Male_____

Age: _____22_____

1. Number of consecutive push-ups = _____30_____

2. Classification = _____good_____ (see table 18.1)

| Worksheet **18.2** | EXTENSION ACTIVITIES |

Name _____   Date _____

1. Given the following data, classify the results of a Push-up Test of Upper-Body Muscular Endurance.

   Gender: _____male_____

   Age: ___34 years___

   Number of consecutive push-ups: _____18_____

   Classification = _____good_____ (see table 18.1)

2. Given the following data, classify the results of a Push-up Test of Upper-Body Muscular Endurance.

   Gender: _____female_____

   Age: ___21 years___

   Number of consecutive push-ups: _____25_____

   Classification = __Very good__ (see table 18.1)

EXTENSION QUESTIONS

1. What are some common mistakes that may occur in administering this lab?

2. Identify possible sources of error in this lab.

3. Assess the practicality of using this lab in the field.

4. Research the reliability and/or validity of this lab using the Internet, journal articles, and other credible sources.

REFERENCES

1. American College of Sports Medicine. *ACSM's Guidelines for Exercise Testing and Prescription,* 7th edition. Philadelphia: Lippincott Williams & Wilkins, 2006, pp. 83–85.

2. Cramer, J. T., and Coburn, J. W. Fitness testing protocols and norms. In *NSCA's Essentials of Personal Training,* eds. R. W. Earle and T. K. Baechle. Champaign, IL: Human Kinetics, 2004.

3. Hoffman, J. *Norms for Fitness, Performance, and Health.* Champaign, IL: Human Kinetics, 2006, pp. 41 and 196.

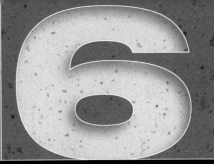

Unit 6

MUSCULAR POWER

Lab 19

40-Yard Dash Test of Speed

BACKGROUND

Speed describes the ability to cover a specific distance as fast as possible. One of the most commonly used tests of speed is the 40-yard dash, and it is often included in a battery of tests for male and female athletes who compete in sports such as football, basketball, volleyball, and baseball.[1,2,3,4] Although it is likely that the original selection of 40 yards for this test was somewhat arbitrary, this distance has now become standard, and many coaches and athletes are familiar with the sprint times associated with this distance.[4]

In this laboratory, you will learn to perform and record the time for the 40-yard dash. You will also learn to estimate the approximate percentile rank associated with 40-yard dash times by gender and age, as well as compare 40-yard dash times with those of athletes in various sports.

KNOW THESE TERMS & ABBREVIATIONS

☐ speed = the ability to cover a specific distance as fast as possible

☐ percentile rank = in this lab, a score between 10% and 90% that shows how the subject performed relative to others in the age group. A percentile ranking of 70, for example, indicates that the subject can run the 40-yard dash faster than 70% of the others in the age group and slower than 30% of the others in the age group.

EQUIPMENT (see Appendix 2 for vendors)   Approximate Price

1. A track or football field or any area of sufficient size
2. Cones, markers, or tape to mark off a distance of
   40 yards on a field or track $10
3. Stopwatch $10

PROCEDURES[4] (see photos 19.1 and 19.2)

1. Typically, the 40-yard dash is performed on a track or football field, but any open area of sufficient size will work.
2. Mark off a distance of 40 yards using cones (on a field) or tape (on a track).
3. Have the subject warm up by jogging (and stretching if desired). After the initial warm-up, the subject should complete four to six intermittent sprints of approximately 10 to 20 yards of 80% to 100% of maximal speed.
4. Have the subject place one or two hands on the starting line of the 40-yard dash (for an example of a four-point stance, see photo 19.1). When ready, the subject starts running as fast as possible. The timer is located

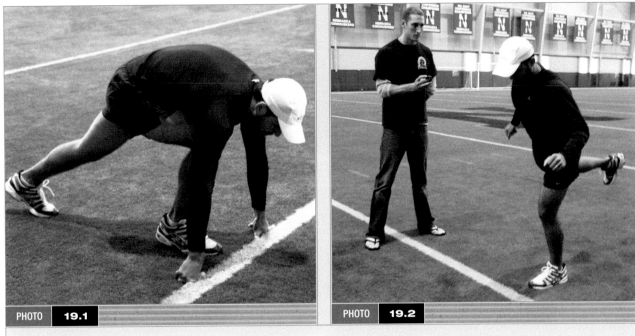

PHOTO 19.1	PHOTO 19.2
Four-point stance at the starting line of the 40-yard dash.	Subject being timed as he crosses the finish line.

at the end line of the 40 yards and begins timing with a stopwatch when the subject's hands leave the starting line. The subject must run as fast as possible for the full 40 yards. The timer stops the stopwatch precisely when the subject crosses the end line (see photo 19.2).

5. The timer records the 40-yard dash time to the nearest 0.01 seconds on worksheet 19.1.

6. Repeat for a total of three trials and select the fastest time. The subject should rest for approximately three minutes (or more) between trials.

7. Table 19.1 provides the percentile ranks for 40-yard dash times in seconds for young males and females (12 to 18 years of age). For college-age subjects, use the percentile ranks in table 19.1 for 16- to 18-year-olds (even though the subject may be older than 18) for the appropriate gender. Table 19.2 provides mean 40-yard dash times in seconds for male and female athletes in selected sports.

Sample Calculation

Name: ___I. M. Fast___

Gender: ___Male___

Age: ___15 years___

40-yard dash time (to the nearest 0.01 seconds):

Trial 1	Trial 2	Trial 3
5.31	5.30	5.24

Fastest trial = ___5.24___ seconds

Approximate percentile rank = ___70___ (see table 19.1)

TABLE	19.1	Percentile ranks for 40-yard dash times in seconds for young (age 12–18) males and females.[4]

	Percentile rank					
	12–13 years		14–15 years		16–18 years	
	Males	Females	Males	Females	Males	Females
90	5.41	5.79	5.02	5.36	4.76	4.93
80	5.63	6.14	5.15	5.68	4.85	5.22
70	5.77	6.49	5.24	6.01	4.90	5.52
60	5.84	6.84	5.32	6.33	4.98	5.82
50	5.97	7.19	5.46	6.65	5.10	6.11
40	6.08	7.54	5.54	6.97	5.13	6.41
30	6.25	7.89	5.78	7.30	5.21	6.71
20	6.32	8.24	6.02	7.62	5.30	7.00
10	6.64	8.59	6.08	7.95	5.46	7.31

TABLE	19.2	Mean (± SD) 40-yard dash times in seconds for male and female athletes in selected sports.[1,2,3,4]

Sport	Gender	Age	$\bar{X} \pm SD$
American football	M	14–15 years	5.40 ± 0.53
American football	M	16–18 years	5.15 ± 0.45
American football	M	College (NCAA Division III)	4.99 ± 0.35
American football	M	College (NCAA Division II)	4.88 ± 0.30
American football	M	College (NCAA Division I)	4.74 ± 0.30
Basketball	M	College (NCAA Division I)	4.81 ± 0.26
Soccer	M	College (NCAA Division III)	4.73 ± 0.18
Ice hockey	F	8–16 years ($\bar{X} \pm SD$ = 12.2 ± 2.1 years)	7.19 ± 0.70
Soccer	F	College (NCAA Division III)	5.34 ± 0.17
Volleyball	F	College (NCAA Division I)	5.62 ± 0.24

| | 40-YARD DASH FORM | Worksheet **19.1** |

Name _____ Date _____

Gender: _____*Male*_____

Age: _____*21*_____

40-yard dash time (to the nearest 0.01 seconds):

| Trial | 1 | 2 | 3 |

5.21   5.20   _____

Fastest trial = ___5.20___ seconds

Percentile rank = ___50___ (see table 19.1)

x 6s sprint

| | EXTENSION ACTIVITIES | Worksheet **19.2** |

Name _____ Date _____

1. Use your own data from the 40-yard dash to determine the approximate percentile rank based on the column in table 19.1 for 16- to 18-year-olds (even though you may be older than 18 years) of your gender.

   40-yard dash time = ___4.85___ seconds
   Approximate percentile rank = ___90___ (see table 19.1)

2. For your gender, which sport and age category in table 19.2 is your 40-yard dash time closest to?

   Sport: ___football___
   Age category: ___18+___

EXTENSION QUESTIONS

1. What are some common mistakes that may occur in administering this lab?
2. Identify possible sources of error in this lab.
3. Assess the practicality of using this lab in the field.
4. Research the reliability and/or validity of this lab using the Internet, journal articles, and other credible sources.

REFERENCES

1. Bracko, M. R., and George J. D. Prediction of ice skating performance with off-ice testing in women's ice hockey players. *J. Strength Cond. Res.* 15: 116–122, 2001.

2. Fry, A. C., Kramer, W. J., Weseman, C. A., Conroy, B. P., Gordon, S. E., Hoffman, J. R., and Maresh, C. M. The effects of an off-season strength and conditioning program on starters and non-starters in women's intercollegiate volleyball. *J. Appl. Sports Sci. Res.* 5: 174–181, 1991.

3. Garstecki, M. A., Latin, R. W., and Cuppett, M. M. Comparison of selected physical fitness and performance variables between NCAA Division I and II football players. *J. Strength Cond. Res.* 18: 292–297, 2004.

4. Hoffman, J. *Norms for Fitness, Performance, and Health.* Champaign, IL: Human Kinetics, 2006, pp. 107–112.

BACKGROUND

Many athletic events involve short, intensive bouts of exercise. The performance of such activities may be limited by the capacity of an individual's anaerobic energy production pathways. Currently, the most popular anaerobic test is the Wingate Anaerobic Test (WanT).[1] This test gauges the energy produced during phosphagen breakdown (ATP–PC system) and anaerobic glycolysis. An athlete's anaerobic work responses can be obtained with a Monark cycle ergometer and the WanT protocol: leg pedaling at maximal effort for 30 seconds against a resistance determined by multiplying the subject's body weight in kg by 0.075. The work performed during the 30-second period is the basis for three important anaerobic indices.

Peak power. Peak power reflects the phosphagen component of anaerobic energy release and indicates the capabilities of the ATP–PC system. It is the greatest work performed during any five-second period (kgm • 5 sec^{-1}) using the following formula:

0.075 kg resistance x kg of body weight

x 6 (the distance in meters traveled by the cycle ergometer flywheel in one revolution)

x greatest number of revolutions of the flywheel in a 5-second period

Mean power. Mean power reflects the glycolytic component (anaerobic glycolysis) plus the phosphagen (ATP–PC system) component of energy release. It is defined as the total work performed during the 30-second test (kgm • 30 sec^{-1}) using the following formula:

0.075 kg resistance x kg of body weight

x 6

x number of revolutions of the flywheel in the 30-second period

Fatigue index. Fatigue index reflects the anaerobic fatigue capabilities of the muscles that are active during cycling. A higher fatigue index indicates a greater proportion of fast twitch muscle fibers. Use the following formula:

$$\frac{\text{greatest work performed in 5-sec period} - \text{lowest work performed in 5-sec period}}{\text{greatest work in 5-sec period}} \times 100$$

KNOW THESE TERMS & ABBREVIATIONS

- BW = body weight
- fatigue index = number reflecting the anaerobic fatigue capabilities of the muscles that are active during cycling
- FFW = fat-free weight
- mean power = the total work performed during the 30-second test (kgm • 30 sec^{-1})

☐ peak power = the greatest work performed during any five-second period (kgm • 5 sec^{-1})

☐ WanT = Wingate Anaerobic Test

☐ W = watts

EQUIPMENT (see Appendix 2 for vendors)	**Approximate Price**
1. Monark cycle ergometer	$2,000
2. Stopwatch	$10

PROCEDURES

Anaerobic work indices will be measured using the WanT on a Monark cycle ergometer equipped with toe clips. Record data from the ergometer on worksheet 20.1.

1. Prior to beginning the test, adjust the seat of the cycle ergometer to allow for near full extension of the subject's legs while pedaling.

2. Warm-up: The WanT will be preceded by a standardized warm-up protocol, which involves pedaling with no resistance for approximately four minutes interspersed with two or three sprints of four to five seconds (see photo 20.1).

3. Following the warm-up period, have the subject begin to pedal with no resistance. At the command "Go," the subject will begin to pedal as fast as possible while the resistance is increased to 0.075 kg per kg of body weight within the first two to three seconds of the test (see photo 20.2).

4. Once the resistance is set, begin the 30-second test. During this time the tester should encourage the subject to give a maximal effort and monitor the resistance setting and elapsed time.

5. Cool-down: After the 30-second test, have the subject continue to pedal for two to three minutes (or longer if the subject desires) with no resistance (see photo 20.3).

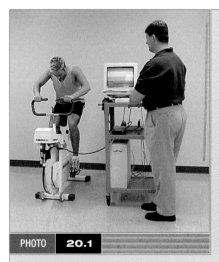

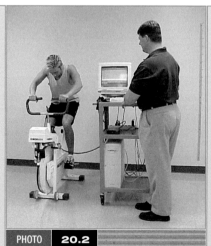

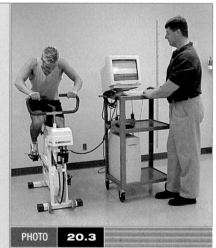

Warm-up prior to the WanT.

At the command "Go," the subject pedals as fast as possible.

Cool-down after the WanT.

Sample Calculations

Gender: _Male_

Body weight: _70 kg_

Fat-free weight: _63 kg_

Resistance = 0.075 × kg of body weight [BW] = 0.075 × 70 kg: _5.25 kg_

Seconds	Resistance	×	6	×	Revolutions	=	Work (kgm • 5 sec^{-1})
0–5	5.25	×	6	×	11	=	346.5
5–10	5.25	×	6	×	12	=	378.0
10–15	5.25	×	6	×	10	=	315.0
15–20	5.25	×	6	×	9	=	283.5
20–25	5.25	×	6	×	9	=	283.5
25–30	5.25	×	6	×	8	=	252.0
0–30	5.25	×	6	×	59	=	1858.5 kgm • 30 sec^{-1}

peak power (PP) = 5.25 kg of resistance × 6 m × 12 revolutions
= 378.0 kgm • 5 sec^{-1} × 12 = 4536.0 kgm • min^{-1} / 6.12 = 741.2 Watts (W)

Percentile rank (see table 20.1) = approximately 64th percentile

PP / BW (W • kgBW^{-1}) = 741.2 / 70 = 10.6 W • kgBW^{-1}

Percentile rank (see table 20.1) = approximately 85th percentile

PP / FFW (W • kgFFW^{-1}) = 741.2 / 63 = 11.8 W • kgFFW^{-1}

Percentile rank (see table 20.1) = approximately 88th percentile

mean power (MP) = 5.25 kg of resistance × 6 m × 59 revolutions
= 1858.5 kgm • 30 sec^{-1} × 2 = 3717 kgm • min^{-1} / 6.12 = 607.4 W

Percentile rank (see table 20.2) = approximately 76th percentile

MP / BW (W • kgBW^{-1}) = 607.4 / 70 = 8.7 W • kgBW^{-1}

Percentile rank (see table 20.2) = approximately 96th percentile

MP / FFW (W • kgFFW^{-1}) = 607.4 / 63 = 9.6 W • kgFFW^{-1}

Percentile rank (see table 20.2) = approximately 99th percentile

$$\text{fatigue index} = \frac{378.0 \text{ kgm • 5 sec}^{-1} - 252.0 \text{ kgm • 5 sec}^{-1}}{378.0 \text{ kgm • 5 sec}^{-1}} \times 100 = 33.33$$

Percentile rank (see table 20.3) = approximately 34th percentile

TABLE	20.1	Percentile norms and descriptive statistics for peak power of the Wingate Anaerobic Test.

Percentile Rank	Watts (W)		$W \cdot kgBW^{-1}$		$W \cdot kgFFW^{-1}$	
	Male	Female	Male	Female	Male	Female
95	866.9	602.1	11.08	9.32	12.26	11.87
90	821.8	560.0	10.89	9.02	11.96	11.47
85	807.1	529.6	10.59	8.92	11.67	11.28
80	776.7	526.6	10.39	8.83	11.47	10.79
75	767.9	517.8	10.39	8.63	11.38	10.69
70	757.1	505.0	10.20	8.53	11.28	10.39
65	744.3	493.3	10.00	8.34	11.08	10.30
60	720.8	479.5	9.80	8.14	10.79	10.10
55	706.1	463.9	9.51	7.85	10.30	9.90
50	689.4	449.1	9.22	7.65	10.20	9.61
45	677.6	447.2	9.02	7.16	10.10	9.41
40	670.8	432.5	8.92	6.96	10.00	8.92
35	661.9	417.8	8.63	6.96	9.90	8.83
30	656.1	399.1	8.53	6.86	9.51	8.73
25	646.3	396.2	8.34	6.77	9.32	8.43
20	617.8	375.6	8.24	6.57	9.12	8.34
15	594.3	361.9	7.45	6.37	8.53	8.04
10	569.8	353.0	7.06	5.98	8.04	7.75
5	530.5	329.5	6.57	5.69	7.45	6.86
M	699.5	454.5	9.18	7.61	10.18	9.54
SD	94.7	81.3	1.43	1.24	1.46	1.51
Maximum	926.7	622.7	11.90	10.64	12.96	12.90
Minimum	500.1	239.3	5.31	4.58	6.55	5.20

Note: BW = body weight, FFW = fat-free weight

Percentile norms and descriptive statistics for mean power of the Wingate Anaerobic Test.   **TABLE   20.2**

Percentile Rank	Watts (W)		W • kgBW^{-1}		W • kgFFW^{-1}	
	Male	Female	Male	Female	Male	Female
95	676.6	483.0	8.63	7.52	9.30	9.43
90	661.8	469.9	8.24	7.31	9.03	9.01
85	630.5	437.0	8.09	7.08	8.88	8.88
80	617.9	419.4	8.01	6.95	8.80	8.76
75	604.3	413.5	7.96	6.93	8.70	8.68
70	600.0	409.7	7.91	6.77	8.63	8.52
65	591.7	402.2	7.70	6.65	8.50	8.32
60	576.8	391.4	7.59	6.59	8.44	8.18
55	574.5	386.0	7.46	6.51	8.24	8.13
50	564.6	381.1	7.44	6.39	8.21	7.93
45	552.8	376.9	7.26	6.20	8.14	7.86
40	547.6	366.9	7.14	6.15	8.04	7.70
35	534.6	360.5	7.08	6.13	7.95	7.57
30	529.7	353.2	7.00	6.03	7.80	7.46
25	520.6	346.8	6.79	5.94	7.64	7.32
20	496.1	336.5	6.59	5.71	7.46	7.11
15	484.6	320.3	6.39	5.56	7.28	7.03
10	470.9	306.1	5.98	5.25	6.83	6.83
5	453.2	286.5	5.56	5.07	6.49	6.70
M	562.7	380.8	7.28	6.35	8.11	7.96
SD	66.5	56.4	0.88	0.73	0.82	0.88
Minimum	441.3	235.4	4.63	4.53	5.72	5.12
Maximum	711.0	528.6	9.07	8.11	9.66	9.66

Note: BW = body weight, FFW = fat-free weight

Reprinted with permission from *Research Quarterly for Exercise and Sport,* Vol. 60, No. 2, pp. 144–151. Copyright © 1989 by the American Alliance for Health, Physical Education, Recreation and Dance, 1900 Association Dr., Reston, VA 20191.

TABLE	20.3	Percentile norms and descriptive statistics for fatigue index.

Percentile Rank	Fatigue Index	
	Male	Female
95	55.0l	48.05
90	51.69	47.33
85	47.40	44.25
80	46.67	43.57
75	44.98	42.19
70	43.51	40.33
65	41.93	39.04
60	39.92	38.21
55	39.48	36.69
50	38.39	35.15
45	36.77	34.36
40	35.04	33.70
35	34.07	30.70
30	31.09	28.74
25	30.23	28.11
20	29.55	26.45
15	26.86	25.00
10	23.18	25.00
5	20.77	19.65
M	37.67	35.05
SD	9.89	8.32
Minimum	14.71	17.86
Maximum	57.51	48.94

Note: N = Males 52, Females 50

Reprinted with permission from *Research Quarterly for Exercise and Sport,* Vol. 60, No. 2, pp. 144–151. Copyright © 1989 by the American Alliance for Health, Physical Education, Recreation and Dance, 1900 Association Dr., Reston, VA 20191.

WINGATE TEST FORM   Worksheet **20.1**

Name _____   *Date* _____

Body weight: _____ kg

Seconds	Resistance	×	6	×	Revolutions	=	Work (kgm • 5 sec⁻¹)
0–5	_____	×	6	×	_____	=	_____
5–10	_____	×	6	×	_____	=	_____
10–15	_____	×	6	×	_____	=	_____
15–20	_____	×	6	×	_____	=	_____
20–25	_____	×	6	×	_____	=	_____
25–30	_____	×	6	×	_____	=	_____
0–30	_____	×	6	×	_____	=	_____ kgm • 30 sec⁻¹

Resistance (0.075 × kg of body weight [BW]) = _____ kg

Peak power = _____ kgm • 5 sec⁻¹ × 12 / 6.12 = _____ Watts

Percentile rank (table 20.1) = _____

Peak power/body weight (W • kgBW⁻¹, table 20.1) = _____

Percentile rank = _____

Peak power/fat-free weight (W • kgFFW⁻¹, table 20.1) = _____

Percentile rank = _____

Mean power = _____ kgm • 30 sec⁻¹ × 2 / 6.12 = _____ Watts

Percentile rank (table 20.2) = _____

Mean power/body weight (W • kgBW⁻¹, table 20.2) = _____

Percentile rank = _____

Mean power/fat-free weight (W • kgFFW⁻¹, table 20.2) = _____

Percentile rank = _____

Fatigue index _____

Percentile rank (table 20.3) = _____

Worksheet 20.2 | EXTENSION ACTIVITIES

Name _____ *Date* _____

1. Mary has a fatigue index of 28.5. What is her percentile rank for fatigue index? Provide a brief interpretation of her fatigue index based on her percentile rank.

2. The 40-yard dash is frequently used to assess football players. Which of the three anaerobic work indices would be best correlated with the 40-yard dash time? Why?

3. Frank Fastwitch (who weighs 175 lbs) performed a Wingate Test, and his results are presented below. Use 0.075 x BW (kg) to determine resistance. Round off resistance to the nearest 0.25 kg.

Seconds	Revolutions
0–5	10
5–10	10
10–15	8
15–20	7
20–25	5
25–30	4

DETERMINE:

A. Peak power _____

B. Mean power _____

C. Fatigue index _____

4. Use your own data to calculate the following:

a. *Peak Power:* Calculate peak power in kgm • 5 sec^{-1} and watts. Report and briefly interpret the absolute (watts) and relative (W • kgBW^{-1}) percentile ranks (table 20.1).

b. *Mean Power:* Calculate mean power in kgm • 30 sec^{-1} and watts. Report and briefly interpret the absolute (watts) and relative (W • kgBW^{-1}) percentile ranks (table 20.2).

c. *Fatigue Index:* Calculate fatigue index and report your percentile rank (table 20.3). What does this imply in terms of how you fatigue in comparison to the rest of the population?

EXTENSION QUESTIONS

1. What are some common mistakes that may occur in administering this lab?

2. Identify possible sources of error in this lab.

3. Assess the practicality of using this lab in the field.

4. Research the reliability and/or validity of this lab using the Internet, journal articles, and other credible sources.

REFERENCES

1. Bar-Or, O. The Wingate Anaerobic Test: An update on methodology, reliability, and validity. *Sports Med.* 4: 381–394, 1987.

2. Maud, P. J., and Schultz, B. B. Norms for the Wingate Anaerobic Test with comparison to another similar test. *Res. Quart. for Exerc. Sport* 60: 144–151, 1989.

Vertical Jump Test for Measuring Muscular Power of the Legs

BACKGROUND

The vertical jump is a commonly used test to assess muscular power of the legs.[1,2,3,4,5,6] Power is defined as (*force* × *distance*) / *time*. Thus, performing the vertical jump and producing great muscular power depend on the ability to produce a high level of force very rapidly. There are two primary ways to test the vertical jump: the squat jump and the countermovement jump. During the squat jump, the subject lowers into the squat position, pauses for a moment, and then jumps vertically as high as possible. During the countermovement jump, the subject starts from a standing position, descends rapidly into a squat position, and then, without stopping at the bottom of the squat, performs a maximal vertical jump. The countermovement jump results in jump heights that are approximately 2 to 4 cm higher than the squat jump.[1] This occurs because there is a rapid transition from the descent (eccentric phase) to the ascent (concentric phase) of the movement. The squat jump, however, tends to result in more reliable scores, presumably due to the variability associated with the countermovement. In addition, muscular power of the legs is more accurately estimated using the squat jump than the countermovement jump.[5]

It is not necessary to use advanced equipment such as a force plate or Vertec device to determine vertical jump height. Vertical jump height can be measured simply by placing chalk on the fingertips of the subject, then having the subject jump next to a wall and touch the wall at the top of the jump. Vertical jump height is measured as the difference between the height of the chalk mark at the level of the highest jump and the height of a chalk mark made while standing with the arm fully extended overhead.

Power output cannot be measured directly from jump height alone, but for the squat jump technique, it can be estimated for both males and females from vertical jump height and body weight using the following regression equation of Sayers et al.:[5]

muscular power (Watts) = (60.7 × vertical jump height (cm))

+ (45.3 × body weight (kg))

− 2055.

Multiple correlation coefficient (R) = 0.94
standard error of estimate (SEE) = 372.9 Watts

In addition, a nomogram has been developed[3] from the equation of Sayers et al.[5] to simplify the estimation of muscular power.

In this laboratory, you will learn to administer the vertical jump test using the squat jump technique and calculate muscular power of the legs from vertical jump height and body weight using the equation of Sayers et al.[5] You will also learn to use the nomogram of Keir et al.[3] to estimate muscular power. You will then compare the subject's vertical jump height in cm and muscular power in Watts to percentile rank norms based on age and gender (tables 21.1–21.4).

Percentile ranks for vertical jump muscular power (Watts) for males by age.[4]

TABLE 21.1

Percentile rank	15–19	20–29	30–39	40–49	50–59	60–69
90	≥4978	≥5676	≥5602	≥5271	≥4841	≥4106
80	4643	5093	4859	4319	4018	3766
70	4506	4882	4685	3992	3703	3466
60	4184	4639	4388	3699	3566	3290
50	4049	4411	4222	3550	3342	3248
40	3857	4296	3966	3241	2937	2842
30	3678	4018	3750	3040	2747	2512
20	3322	3774	3484	2707	2511	2382
10	2908	3456	2764	2511	2080	1636
<10	<2908	<3456	<2764	<2511	<2080	<1636

Note: The percentile ranks in this table are for the squat jump technique.

Percentile ranks for vertical jump muscular power (Watts) for females by age.[4]

TABLE 21.2

Percentile rank	15–19	20–29	30–39	40–49	50–59	60–69
90	≥3514	≥3667	≥3581	≥2989	≥2742	≥2604
80	3166	3249	3192	2674	2558	2474
70	2945	3007	2844	2503	2470	1779
60	2794	2803	2549	2287	2160	1717
50	2590	2628	2388	2157	1956	1465
40	2398	2477	2334	2100	1700	1316
30	2280	2374	2258	1824	1497	1262
20	2155	2270	2146	1687	1385	1197
10	1878	1971	1692	1330	1006	570
<10	<1878	<1971	<1692	<1330	<1006	<570

Note: The percentile ranks in this table are for the squat jump technique.

| TABLE | 21.3 | Percentile ranks for vertical jump height (cm) for males by age.[4] |

Percentile rank	15–19	20–29	30–39	40–49	50–59	60–69
90	≥57	≥60	≥54	≥51	≥47	≥34
80	55	57	51	42	40	32
70	53	55	48	38	36	30
60	50	53	45	35	34	28
50	47	50	42	33	30	26
40	45	47	39	31	27	24
30	43	44	36	29	24	22
20	41	41	30	25	17	17
10	38	38	23	21	10	12
<10	<38	<38	<23	<21	<10	<12

Note: The percentile ranks in this table are for the squat jump technique.

| TABLE | 21.4 | Percentile ranks for vertical jump height (cm) for females by age.[4] |

Percentile rank	15–19	20–29	30–39	40–49	50–59	60–69
90	≥41	≥40	≥37	≥32	≥26	≥20
80	39	37	35	30	24	18
70	37	35	33	28	22	16
60	35	33	31	26	20	14
50	33	30	29	24	18	12
40	31	28	27	22	15	10
30	29	26	25	20	12	8
20	27	24	23	17	9	6
10	25	19	19	14	5	3
<10	<25	<19	<19	<14	<5	<3

Note: The percentile ranks in this table are for the squat jump technique.

KNOW THESE TERMS & ABBREVIATIONS

☐ maximal effort vertical jump = total jump height

☐ nomogram = a graph that shows the relationship between variables. In this case, the nomogram shows the relationship between vertical jump height, body weight, and muscular power in Watts.

☐ power = (force × distance) / time

☐ R = multiple correlation coefficient, a numerical measure of how well a dependent variable can be predicted from a combination of independent variables (a number between –0 and 1)

☐ SEE = standard error of estimate, a measure of the accuracy of predictions made using a regression equation

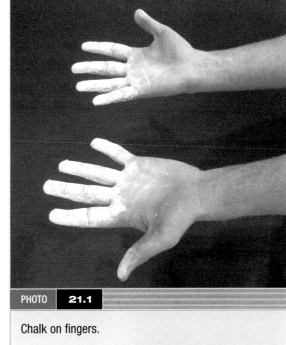

PHOTO **21.1**

Chalk on fingers.

EQUIPMENT
(see Appendix 2 for vendors)

	Approximate Price
1. Scale	$175 or less
2. Meter stick	$10
3. Chalk	$5

PROCEDURES (see photos 21.1 to 21.4)

1. Measure the subject's body weight (kg) and record it on worksheet 21.1.

2. Measure the subject's standing reach height by putting chalk on the person's fingertips (photo 21.1) and having him or her stand next to a wall, reach as high as possible, and touch the wall (photo 21.2). The distance between the floor and the chalk mark on the wall is the standing reach height. Record the standing reach height on worksheet 21.1.

3. Have the subject perform a general warm-up of jogging or cycle ergometry for five minutes and three to five practice jumps at approximately 50% of maximal capability.

4. Place chalk on the fingertips prior to each maximal effort vertical jump.

5. Have the subject assume a squat position with the knees at approximately 90 degrees[5] and then pause for one to two seconds prior to initiating a maximal vertical jump (photo 21.3). The feet should be approximately shoulder-width apart and the dominant arm should be toward the wall. The arms should be positioned posterior to the torso so that they can be thrust upward during the jump. The subject should perform at least three maximal effort vertical jumps or continue until a plateau in performance is achieved. Provide at least one minute of rest between attempts.[6] Record the height (from the floor to the chalk mark) of each maximal effort vertical jump (photo 21.4; called the total jump height) on worksheet 21.1.

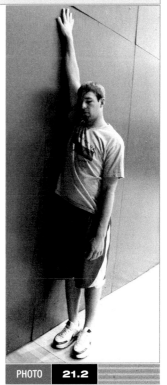

PHOTO **21.2**

Standing reach height.

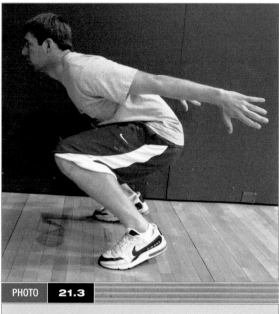

PHOTO   21.3

Squat position prior to initiating a maximal vertical jump.

6. Calculate the vertical jump height, defined as the difference in cm between the total jump height and the standing reach height (vertical jump height = total jump height – standing reach height; see worksheet 21.1).

7. Calculate muscular power using the equation of Sayers et al.[5] based on the subject's best vertical jump height and body weight (see sample calculation below). Alternatively, muscular power can be estimated using the nomogram of Keir et al.,[3] which is derived from the equation of Sayers et al.[5] (see sample estimation given in figure 21.1).

8. Compare the subject's vertical jump height in cm and muscular power in Watts to the percentile rank norms in tables 21.1 through 21.4.[4] These percentile rank norms are for the squat jump technique only and cannot be used for the countermovement jump technique.

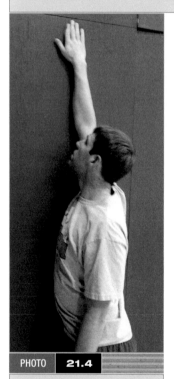

PHOTO   21.4

Touch the chalked fingers to the wall at the highest point of the maximal vertical jump.

Sample Calculations

Name: __I. M. Powerful__

Gender: ___Male___

Body Weight: ___81.6 kg___

Height: ___153 cm___

Age: ___21 years___

standing reach height ___205___ cm

total jump height # 1 ___243___ cm

   total jump height – standing reach height = vertical jump height

   ___243___ cm – ___205___ cm = ___38___ cm

total jump height # 2 ___245___ cm

   total jump height – standing reach height = vertical jump height

   ___245___ cm – ___205___ cm = ___(40)___ cm

total jump height # 3 ___244___ cm

   total jump height – standing reach height = vertical jump height

   ___244___ cm – ___205___ cm = ___39___ cm

muscular power = (60.7 × ___40___ cm) + (45.3 × ___81.6___ kg) – 2055 = ___(4069)___ Watts

estimated muscular power from the nomogram (see figure 21.1) = ___4050___ Watts

percentile rank based on muscular power (Watts) ___32nd percentile___ (see table 21.1)

percentile rank based on vertical jump height (cm) ___18th percentile___ (see table 21.3)

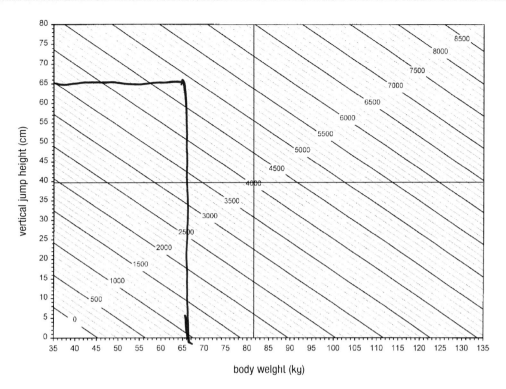

To estimate muscular power (Watts) from the vertical jump height and body weight, first draw a vertical line upward from the x-axis at a point equal to the subject's body weight (kg). Next, draw a horizontal line to the right from the y-axis at a level equal to the subject's best vertical jump height (cm). Find the muscular power value (expressed in Watts) that is closest to the intersection of the two lines.[3] For example, based on the data provided in the sample calculations (body weight = 81.6 kg and best vertical jump height = 40 cm), the estimated muscular power is approximately 4050 Watts.

Worksheet **21.1**   DETERMINATION OF VERTICAL JUMP HEIGHT AND MUSCULAR POWER

Name _____   Date _____

Gender: ___Male_____

Age: ___21_____

Body weight:: ___65.8_____ kg

Height:: ___5'8_____ cm

Age: ___21_____

standing reach height ___-1_____ cm

total jump height # 1 ___25_____ cm

total jump height − standing reach height = vertical jump height

___65_____ cm − ___-1_____ cm = ___64_____ cm

total jump height # 2 ___26_____ cm

total jump height − standing reach height = vertical jump height

___66_____ cm − ___1_____ cm = ___65_____ cm

total jump height # 3 _____ cm

total jump height − standing reach height = vertical jump height

_____ cm − _____ cm = _____ cm

muscular power = (60.7 × ___26___ cm) + (45.3 × ___65.8___ kg) − 2055 = ___2,443.24___ Watts

estimated muscular power from the nomogram (see figure 21.2) = ___2500_____ Watts

percentile rank based on muscular power (see tables 21.1 and 21.2) ___90%___ Watts

percentile rank based on vertical jump height (see tables 21.3 and 21.4) ___95%___ cm

$(60.7 \times 25) + (45.3 \times 65.8) - 2055$

$1,517.5 + 2,980.74 - 2055$

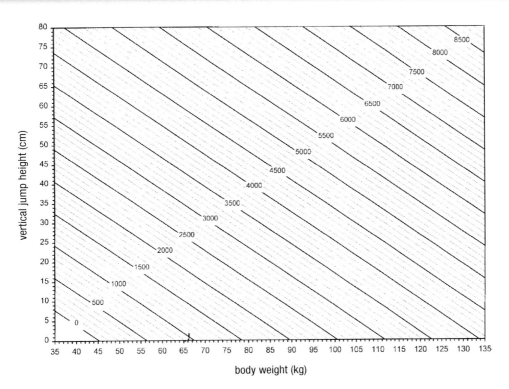

To estimate muscular power (Watts) from the vertical jump height and body weight, first draw a vertical line upward from the x-axis at a point equal to the subject's body weight (kg). Next, draw a horizontal line to the right from the y-axis at a level equal to the subject's best vertical jump height (cm). Find the muscular power value (expressed in Watts) that is closest to the intersection of the two lines.[3]

Worksheet **21.2** | EXTENSION ACTIVITIES

Name _____   *Date* _____

Gender: _____ Female _____

Age: _____ 26 years _____

Body weight: _____ 54 _____ kg

Vertical jump height: _____ 30 _____ cm

muscular power = (60.7 × _____ 30 _____ cm) + (45.3 × _____ 54 _____ kg) – 2055 = _____ 2212 _____ Watts

estimated muscular power from the nomogram (see figure 21.2) = _____ 2300 _____ Watts

percentile rank based on muscular power (table 21.2) _____ 90 _____ Watts

percentile rank based on vertical jump height (table 21.4) _____ 90 _____ cm

EXTENSION QUESTIONS

1. What are some common mistakes that may occur in administering this lab?
2. Identify possible sources of error in this lab.
3. Assess the practicality of using this lab in the field.
4. Research the reliability and/or validity of this lab using the Internet, journal articles, and other credible sources.

REFERENCES

1. Bobbert, M. F., and Casius, J. R. Is the effect of a countermovement on jump height due to active state development? *Med. Sci. Sports Exerc.* 37: 440–446, 2005.

2. Burkett, L. N., Phillips, W. T., and Ziuraitis, J. The best warm up for the vertical jump in college-age athletic men. *J. Strength Cond. Res.* 19: 673–676, 2005.

3. Keir, P. J., Jamnik, V. K., and Gledhill, N. Technical-methodological report: A nomogram for peak leg power in the vertical jump. *J. Strength Cond. Res.* 17: 701–703, 2003.

4. Payne, N., Gledhill, N., Katzmarzyk, P. T., Jamnik, V. K., and Keir, J. P. Canadian musculoskeletal fitness norms. *Can. J. of Appl. Physiol.* 25: 430–442, 2000.

5. Sayers, S. P., Harackiewicz, D. V., Harman, E. A., Frykman, P. N., and Rosenstein, M. T. Cross validation of three jump power equations. *Med. Sci. Sports Exerc.* 31: 572–577, 1999.

6. Stockbrugger, B. A., and Haennel, R. G. Contributing factors to performance of a medicine ball explosive power test: A comparison between jump and nonjump athletes. *J. Strength Cond. Res.* 17: 768–774, 2003.

Standing Long Jump Test

BACKGROUND

The standing long jump is a test of muscular power (power = (force × distance) / time) of the legs and conceptually is similar to the vertical jump test. The standing long jump, however, involves jumping horizontally as far as possible, whereas the vertical jump test measures the height that the subject can jump. The standing long jump distance is highly correlated with other indices of muscular power, such as mean and peak power from the Wingate test (see Lab 20) and jumping height from the vertical jump test (see Lab 21).[2,6]

KNOW THESE TERMS & ABBREVIATIONS

☐ mean power = the total work performed (kgm • 30 sec^{-1}) during the 30-second Wingate test (see Lab 20)

☐ peak power = the greatest work performed (kgm • 5 sec^{-1}) during any five-second period of the Wingate test (see Lab 20)

☐ power = (force × distance) / time

EQUIPMENT (see Appendix 2 for vendors)   Approximate Price

Tape measure $10

PROCEDURES

1. Have the subject perform a generalized warm-up.

2. Position the subject facing the starting line with feet parallel and shoulder-width apart (see photo 22.1).

3. Have the subject simultaneously drop into a squat position to a knee joint angle of about 90 degrees and thrust the arms backward behind the torso (see photo 22.2). A knee joint angle of 90 degrees allows force to be applied to the floor for a longer period of time than a knee joint angle of 45 degrees and, therefore, results in a jumping distance that is typically about 25 cm farther.[8] Many people appear to be less powerful than they really are in this test because they do not effectively coordinate the leg and arm motions. It is important for subjects to keep this in mind as they follow the procedures.

4. At the bottom of the squat (a knee joint angle of 90 degrees), have the subject rapidly transition to a jumping motion using both feet simultaneously. During the jumping motion, the subject should swing the arms and legs forward. Powerful arm swings can add 16–21% to the jumping distance.[1,7,8]

5. Have the subject land on both feet together simultaneously (see photo 22.3).

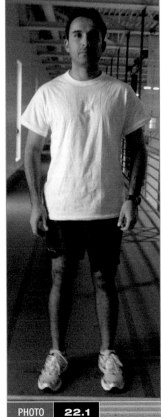

PHOTO   **22.1**

Facing the starting line with feet parallel and shoulder-width apart.

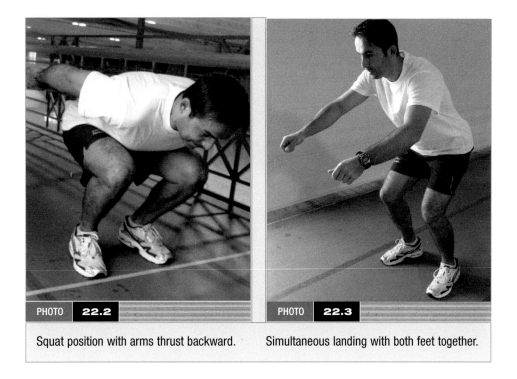

PHOTO 22.2	PHOTO 22.3
Squat position with arms thrust backward.	Simultaneous landing with both feet together.

6. Have the subject perform at least three practice standing long jumps and at least three recorded standing long jumps. The subject should continue the jumps as long as scores increase.

7. Record the jumping distance from the starting line to the more rearward of the two heels on worksheet 22.1.

8. Discard an attempt if the subject falls backward.

9. Compare the subject's best standing long jump distance in cm to the percentile rank norms in table 22.1 and the mean values for various samples in table 22.2.

Percentile ranks for the standing long jump distance (cm) for college age (17+ years of age) males and females.[3]		TABLE 22.1

Percentile rank	Males	Females
95	257	206
75	236	183
50	218	165
25	198	150
5	160	124

TABLE 22.2	Age, height, body weight, and standing long jump distances (mean ± SD) for various athletic and non-athletic samples.			

Athlete	Age (years)	Height (cm)	Body weight (kg)	Jump distance (cm)
Division 1 football players (all positions)[6]	21 ± 1	N/A	98.2 ± 16.4	268 ± 21
Division 1 football players (backs)[6]	21 ± 1	N/A	83.8 ± 6.1	284 ± 16
Division 1 football players (linebackers)[6]	21 ± 1	N/A	99.3 ± 3.9	271 ± 9
Division 1 football players (linemen)[6]	20 ± 1	N/A	117.0 ± 11.4	250 ± 19
Taiwanese college students (female)[8]	20 ± 1	160 ± 6	50.7 ± 10.8	93 ± 20
Untrained men[4]	31 ± 4	178 ± 6	75.0 ± 7.3	215 ± 23
Undergraduate kinesiology students (male)[5]	22 ± 3	179 ± 7	82.7 ± 15.5	227 ± 21

Sample Calculations

Name: _Stan D. Long-Jump_

Gender: _male_

Age: _21 years_

Standing Long Jump Distance #1 _191_ cm

Standing Long Jump Distance #2 _198_ cm

Standing Long Jump Distance #3 _202_ cm

Standing Long Jump Distance #4 _(204)_ cm

Standing Long Jump Distance #5 _200_ cm

Standing Long Jump Distance #6 _____ cm

Standing Long Jump Distance #7 _____ cm

Percentile rank = _32_ (see table 22.1)

STANDING LONG JUMP TEST   Worksheet **22.1**

Name _____   Date _____

Gender: _____Male_____

Age: _____21_____

Standing Long Jump Distance #1 _____260_____ cm

Standing Long Jump Distance #2 _____270_____ cm

Standing Long Jump Distance #3 _____ cm

Standing Long Jump Distance #4 _____ cm

Standing Long Jump Distance #5 _____ cm

Standing Long Jump Distance #6 _____ cm

Standing Long Jump Distance #7 _____ cm

Percentile rank = _____95%_____ (see table 22.1)

Worksheet 22.2   EXTENSION ACTIVITIES

Name _____   *Date* _____

1. On the blank graph below, draw the expected relationship between age and standing long jump distance.

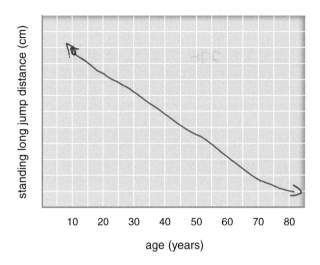

2. Sally jumps 185 cm and John jumps 200 cm during the standing long jump test. Use table 22.1 to determine their approximate percentile ranks.

   Sally: _____~~5~~ 25_____ percentile rank

   John: _____75_____ percentile rank

EXTENSION QUESTIONS

1. What are some common mistakes that may occur in administering this lab?

2. Identify possible sources of error in this lab.

3. Assess the practicality of using this lab in the field.

4. Research the reliability and/or validity of this lab using the Internet, journal articles, and other credible sources.

REFERENCES

1. Ashby, B. M., and Heegaard, J. H. Role of arm motion in the standing long jump. *J. Biomech.* 35: 1631–1637, 2002.

2. Izquierdo, M., Aguado, X., Gonzalez, R., Lopez, J. L., and Hakkinen, K. Maximal and explosive force production capacity and balance performance in men of different ages. *Eur. J. Appl. Physiol.* 79: 260–267, 1999.

3. Johnson, B. L., and Nelson, J. K. *Practical Measurements for Evaluation in Physical Education.* Edina, MN: Burgess Publishing, 1986, p. 213.

4. Moriss, C. J., Tolfrey, K., and Coppack, R. J. Effects of short-term isokinetic training on standing long-jump performance in untrained men. *J. Strength Cond. Res.* 15: 498–502, 2001.

5. Murray, D. P., Brown, L. E., Zinder, S. M., Noffal, G. J., Bera, S. G., and Garrett, N. M. Effects of velocity-specific training on rate of velocity development, peak torque, and performance. *J. Strength Cond. Res.* 21: 870–874, 2007.

6. Seiler, S., Taylor, M., Diana, R., Layes, J., Newton, P., and Brown, B. Assessing anaerobic power in collegiate football players. *J. Appl. Sport Sci. Res.* 4: 9–15, 1990.

7. Wakai, M., and Linthorne, N. P. Optimum take-off angle in the standing long jump. *Human Move. Sci.* 24: 81–96, 2005.

8. Wu, W.-L. Wu, J.-H., Lin, H.-T., and Wang, G. J. Biomechanical analysis of the standing long jump. *Biomed. Eng.* 15: 186–192, 2003.

Backward, Overhead Medicine Ball Throw Test of Total Body Power

BACKGROUND

The backward, overhead medicine ball (BOMB) throw is a test of total body power. Both upper-body and lower-body power contribute to the distance the medicine ball can be thrown.[4] While the test is designed to assess total body power, to date there is no equation that can be used to estimate power output (expressed in Watts) from the distance the medicine ball is thrown. Rather, it is assumed that longer distances are associated with greater muscular power output. Recent studies have shown that the distance the medicine ball is thrown is correlated with other indices of muscular power, such as the vertical jump.[2,3,4]

The BOMB throwing technique involves: (1) taking the medicine ball in both hands with the arms fully extended; (2) bending at the knees (squatting) until the ball reaches approximately the level of the knees; and (3) standing up quickly to throw the medicine ball backward over the top of the head as far as possible.[2] To maximize distance, the subject should perform the motion as fast as possible. The throwing motion is similar to a vertical jump and, in some cases, the subject may come off the ground when performing the test.

In this laboratory, you will learn to administer the BOMB throw test. You will then compare the distance the medicine ball is thrown to values for male and female athletes from various sports (table 23.1).

| TABLE 23.1 | Data for the BOMB throw test for selected male and female athletes. |

Athlete	Age (years)	Height (m)	Weight (kg)	Medicine ball weight (kg)	Throw distance (m)
Volleyball players (male and female)[3]	22.8 ± 3.7	N/A	75.7 ± 14.8	3	12.59 ± 3.31
Wrestlers (male)[4]	20.0 ± 2.9	1.74 ± 0.07	84.8 ± 25.3	3	14.2 ± 1.8
Volleyball players (male)[4]	18.9 ± 1.4	1.89 ± 0.07	82.3 ± 8.9	3	15.4 ± 1.1
Football players (male)[2]	20.6 ± 1.3	1.83 ± 5.6	102.8 ± 19.4	7	10.41 ± 1.45

Note: Values are mean ± standard deviation.

KNOW THESE TERMS & ABBREVIATIONS

☐ power = (force × distance) / time

☐ total body power = a combination of upper- and lower-body power ((force × distance) / time) output. Total body power is assessed using the distance that the medicine ball can be thrown.

EQUIPMENT (see Appendix 2 for vendors)	Approximate Price
1. 3-kg medicine ball	$29–$35
2. Tape measure	$7–$29

PROCEDURES[4]

1. Have the subject perform a generalized warm-up.

2. Position the subject facing away from the area where the medicine ball will be thrown (see photo 23.1).

3. Have the subject grasp the medicine ball with both hands, with arms extended and perpendicular to the ground (see photo 23.2).

4. Space the subject's heels slightly wider than the shoulders so the arms and medicine ball will have room to swing between the knees during the throw (see photo 23.2).

5. For each throw, have the subject rapidly descend into a squatting position. As the subject descends into the squatting position, the elbows should be kept extended. The ball should swing backward between the legs (see photo 23.3).

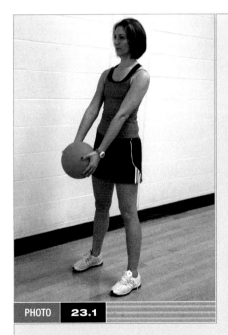

PHOTO **23.1**

Starting position for the BOMB throw test.

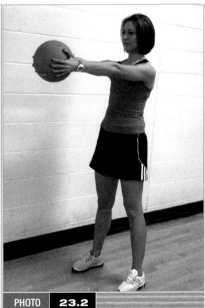

PHOTO **23.2**

Grasping the medicine ball, with both hands extended and perpendicular to the ground.

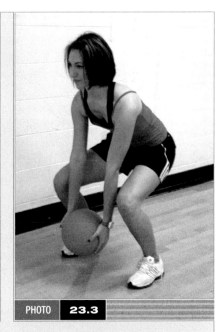

PHOTO **23.3**

The subject in squatting position with the elbows extended.

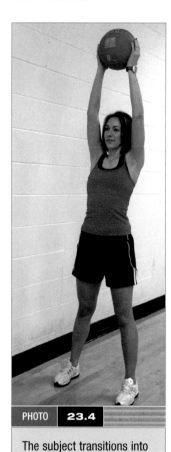

The subject transitions into
the upward motion of the
throw.

6. At the bottom of the squat, the subject should, without stopping, transition into the upward motion of the throw (photo 23.4). This upward motion is similar to that of a vertical jump, with the addition that the subject throws the medicine ball backward over the head. During the throw, the subject should try to keep the arms straight and use a "pendulum action" to maximize throwing distance.[3]

7. After each throw, measure the distance from between the subject's feet and the point where the medicine ball makes first contact with the ground or floor.

8. Repeat until three consecutive throws are within 0.50 meters of the best throw.[4] This will typically take up to six trials.[1] Provide at least one minute of rest between trials.[4] Record the distance of each throw on worksheet 23.1. The longest throw is selected as the subject's score.

Sample Calculation

Name: _John Doe_

Gender: _male_

Body weight: _81.6_ kg

Height: _153_ cm

Age: _21 years_

Throwing Distance #1 _12.1_ m

Throwing Distance #2 _12.7_ m

Throwing Distance #3 _13.2_ m

Throwing Distance #4 _(13.4)_ m

Throwing Distance #5 _13.3_ m

Throwing Distance #6 _____ m

BACKWARD OVERHEAD MEDICINE BALL THROW TEST | Worksheet **23.1**

Name _____   Date _____

Gender: ___Male_____

Body weight: ___14s_____ kg

Height: ___5'4_____ cm

Age: ___21_____ years

Throwing Distance #1 ___12.2_____ m

Throwing Distance #2 ___13.3_____ m

Throwing Distance #3 _____ m

Throwing Distance #4 _____ m

Throwing Distance #5 _____ m

Throwing Distance #6 _____ m

EXTENSION ACTIVITIES | Worksheet **23.2**

Name _____   Date _____

1. On the blank graph below, draw the expected relationship between the BOMB throw distance and vertical jump power in a sample of basketball players. Briefly explain your graph.

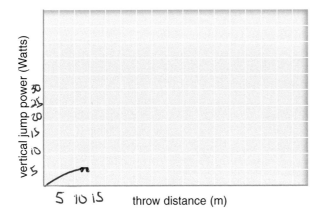

2. Which of the following activities would most likely be correlated with the BOMB throw distance? Briefly explain your selection.

   a. maximal bench press strength

   b. 400-meter sprint time

   c. standing long jump

   d. pull-ups

EXTENSION QUESTIONS

1. What are some common mistakes that may occur in administering this lab?

2. Identify possible sources of error in this lab.

3. Assess the practicality of using this lab in the field.

4. Research the reliability and/or validity of this lab using the Internet, journal articles, and other credible sources.

REFERENCES

1. Duncan, M. J., Al-Nakeeb, Y., and Nevill, A. M. Influence of familiarization on a backward, overhead medicine ball explosive power test. *Res. Sports Med.* 13: 345–352, 2005.

2. Mayhew, J. L., Bird, M., Cole, M. L., Koch, A. J., Jacques, J. A., Ware, J. S., Buford, B. N., and Fletcher, K. M. Comparison of the backward overhead medicine ball throw to power production in college football players. *J. Strength Cond. Res.* 19: 514–518, 2005.

3. Stockbrugger, B. A., and Haennel, R. G. Validity and reliability of a medicine ball explosive power test. *J. Strength Cond. Res.* 15: 431–438, 2001.

4. Stockbrugger, B. A., and Haennel, R. G. Contributing factors to performance of a medicine ball explosive power test: A comparison between jump and nonjump athletes. *J. Strength Cond. Res.* 17: 768–774, 2003.

Unit 7

BODY COMPOSITION AND BODY BUILD

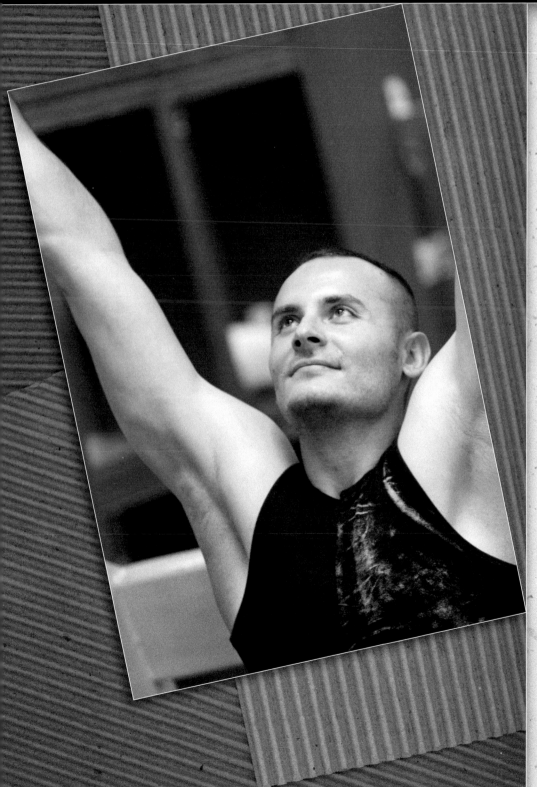

BACKGROUND

Laboratory methods for body composition assessment represent the most accurate means available for determining the amount of fat and fat-free tissue in live subjects. Generally, underwater weighing is considered the "gold standard" for determining body composition characteristics. Often, however, underwater weighing is not practical for assessing large groups of subjects in field situations.

Assessment of body composition by skinfold measurements is a simple and relatively accurate method that requires minimal equipment and can be used with large numbers of subjects in a field setting. Skinfold measurements can be used in multiple regression "prediction" equations to estimate body composition (body density [DB], percent fat [% fat], fat-free weight [FFW], fat weight [FW]). The results of skinfold methods to determine body composition are usually within 3% to 5% of underwater weighing.

The ability to predict body composition from skinfolds is simply based on the fact that fat or fat-free tissues accumulate in relatively predictable patterns in similarly aged individuals of the same gender. Therefore, if specific sites are measured, the measurements will be influenced by the amount of the individual's adipose or fat-free tissue.

In this laboratory the technique for skinfold measurement will be outlined, and you will use the measurements to predict various aspects of body composition.

KNOW THESE TERMS & ABBREVIATIONS

- [ ] DB = body density
- [ ] FFW = fat-free weight
- [ ] FW = fat weight
- [ ] % fat = percent fat

EQUIPMENT (see Appendix 2 for vendors)

	Approximate Price
1. Tape measure	$7–$29
2. Skinfold calipers	$150–$480

PROCEDURES[2]

1. Measure and mark the anatomical sites with a marker (see sites below in photos 24.1 through 24.13). Three sites are to be measured for each gender. Both males and females are measured at the thigh site. Males are also measured at the chest and abdomen, females at the triceps and suprailium.

2. Take all measurements on the right side of the body.

3. Grasp the skinfold of the subject firmly with the thumb and forefinger and pull away from the body.

4. Hold the caliper perpendicular to the skinfold. The caliper should be approximately 1 cm away from the thumb and forefinger so that the pressure of the caliper will not be affected.

5. Read the skinfold size approximately one to two seconds after the caliper thumb grip has been released.

6. Take three measurements per site at least 15 seconds apart to allow the skinfold site to return to normal. If the repeated measurements vary by more than 1 mm, more measurements should be taken. Use the mean of the recorded measurements that are within 1 mm as the representative skinfold value in the equation.

7. Calculate body composition characteristics using worksheet 24.1.

Equations

Males (ages 18–61 years)[3]

DB = 1.1093800 − (0.0008267 (X_2)) + (0.0000016 $(X_2)^2$) − (0.0002574 (X_4)))

R = 0.91

SEE = 0.008 kg • L^{-1}

X_2 = sum of chest, abdomen, and thigh skinfolds in mm

X_4 = age in years

Females (ages 18–55 years)[3]

DB = 1.099421 − (0.0009929 (X_3)) + (0.0000023 $(X_3)^2$) − (0.0001392 (X_4)))

R = 0.84

SEE = 0.009 kg • L^{-1}

X_3 = sum of triceps, thigh, and suprailium skinfolds in mm

X_4 = age in years

SEE = standard error of estimate, R = multiple correlation coefficient

% fat = (((4.57 / DB) − 4.142) × 100)[1]

fat weight = body weight × (% fat/100)

fat-free weight = body weight − fat weight

body weight goal = FFW / (1 − (Target % fat / 100))

Sample Calculations

Gender: _Male_

Body weight: _80.0 kg_

Age: _25 years_

Sum of chest, abdomen, and thigh skinfolds: _40 mm_

DB = 1.1093800 − (0.0008267 (40)) + (0.0000016 (40)^2) − (0.0002574 (25))

DB = 1.1093800 − 0.03307 + 0.00256 − 0.006435 = 1.0724 kg • L^{-1}

% fat = ((4.57 / 1.0724) − 4.142) × 100 = 11.9 % fat

fat weight = 80.0 × (11.9 / 100) = 9.5 kg

fat-free weight = 80.0 − 9.5 = 70.5 kg

body weight goal of 8.0 % fat = 70.5 / (1 − (8.0 / 100)) = 76.6 kg

Gender: _Female_

Body weight: _65 kg_

Age: _30 years_

Sum of triceps, thigh, and suprailium skinfolds: _55 mm_

DB = 1.099421 − (0.0009929 (55)) + (0.0000023 (55)^2) − 0.0001392 (30)

DB = 1.099421 − 0.05461 + 0.00696 − 0.004176 = 1.0476

% fat = ((4.57 / 1.0476) − 4.142) × 100 = 22.0 % fat

fat weight = 65 × (22.0 / 100) = 14.3 kg

fat-free weight = 65 − 14.3 = 50.7 kg

body weight goal of 15.0 % fat = 50.7 / (1 − (15.0 / 100)) = 59.6 kg

Skinfold Sites[3]

CHEST (see photos 24.1–24.3): a diagonal fold taken one half of the distance between the anterior axillary line and the nipple (males).

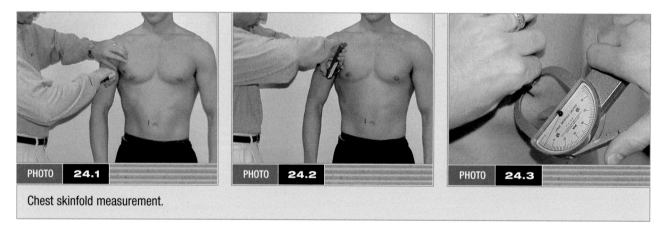

| PHOTO 24.1 | PHOTO 24.2 | PHOTO 24.3 |

Chest skinfold measurement.

ABDOMEN (see photos 24.4–24.6): a vertical fold taken at a lateral distance of approximately 2 cm from the umbilicus (males).

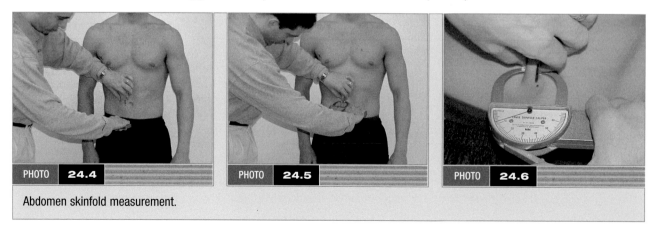

| PHOTO 24.4 | PHOTO 24.5 | PHOTO 24.6 |

Abdomen skinfold measurement.

THIGH (see photos 24.7–24.9): a vertical fold on the anterior aspect of the thigh, midway between hip and knee joints (males and females).

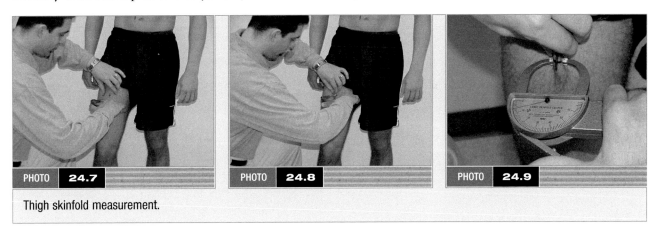

Thigh skinfold measurement.

TRICEPS (see photos 24.10–24.12): a vertical fold on the posterior midline of the upper arm, halfway between the acromion and olecranon processes; the elbow should be extended and relaxed (females).

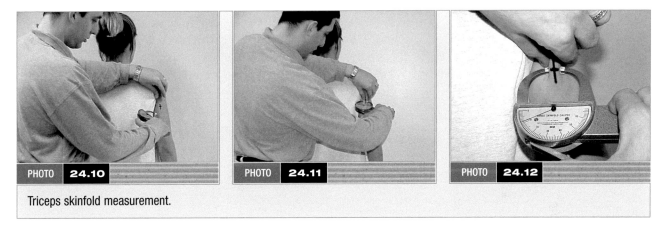

Triceps skinfold measurement.

SUPRAILIUM (see photos 24.13–24.15): a diagonal fold above the crest of the ilium at the spot where an imaginary line would come down from the anterior axillary line (females).

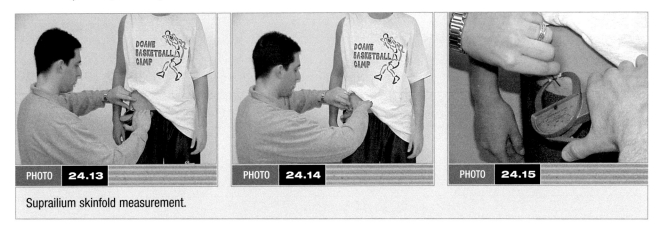

Suprailium skinfold measurement.

Note: For accurate measures, do not take measurements when the skin is wet, immediately after exercise, or when the subject is overheated.

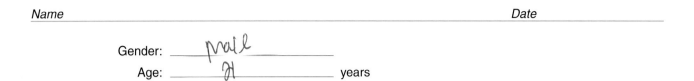

Worksheet 24.1 — SKINFOLD ESTIMATIONS OF BODY COMPOSITION

Name _____   Date _____

Gender: _____ Male _____

Age: _____ 21 _____ years

Body weight: _____ kg

Skinfold Measurements (mm)

	Trial 1	Trial 2	Trial 3	Mean
Triceps				
Suprailium				
Abdomen	9	9		
Thigh ✗	17	17		
Chest	14.5	14.5		

Sum of chest, abdomen, and thigh skinfolds = _____ 81 _____

Sum of triceps, thigh, and suprailium skinfolds = _____

Use the gender-specific equations on p. 165 to calcualte DB.

DB = _____ $kg \cdot L^{-1}$

Use the equations on p. 165 to calculate % fat, FW, and FFW.

% fat = _____ %   FW = _____ kg   FFW = _____ kg

Worksheet 24.2 — EXTENSION ACTIVITIES

Name _____   Date _____

1. A subject's % fat, determined by skinfolds, was estimated to be 16.9% (DB = 1.0600 $kg \cdot L^{-1}$). If the SEE of the predicted body density value is equal to 0.0050 $kg \cdot L^{-1}$, then this subject's % fat is likely to fall between what two values?

2. List potential sources of error when estimating body composition from skinfold equations.

   Water Weight, Machine Error.

3. Using the skinfold prediction equations on page 165, calculate your body density and convert this value to % fat.

EXTENSION QUESTIONS

1. What are some common mistakes that may occur in administering this lab?

2. Assess the practicality of using this lab in the field.

3. Research the reliability and/or validity of this lab using the Internet, journal articles, and other credible sources.

REFERENCES

1. Brozek, J., Grande, F., Anderson, J. T., and Keys, A. Densitometric analysis of body composition: Revision of some quantitative assumptions. *Ann. N.Y. Acad. Sci.* 110: 113–140, 1963.

2. Harrison, G. G., Buskirk, E. R., Carter, J. E. L., Johnston, F. E., Lohman, T. G., Pollock, M. L., Roche, A. F., and Wilmore, J. Skinfold thicknesses and measurement techniques. In *Anthropometric Standardization Reference Manual,* eds. T. G. Lohman, A. F. Roche, and R. Martorell. Champaign, IL: Human Kinetics, pp. 55–70, 1988.

3. Jackson, A. S., and Pollock, M. L. Practical assessment of body composition. *Physician Sportsmed.* 13: 76–90, 1985.

BACKGROUND

Three primary anthropometric-based parameters that can provide information regarding the risk of developing cardiovascular disease, type 2 diabetes, dyslipidemia, obesity, and/or hypertension are: body mass index (BMI), waist-to-hip ratio, and waist circumference.[1,3,4,5,8] Each of these parameters can be used to classify individuals with regard to their health risk. In addition, they are commonly used in epidemiological studies because they are associated with various diseases and risk factors, require few measurements, and are simple to calculate.

In this laboratory, the techniques and landmarks for measuring height and body weight, as well as waist 1, waist 2, and hips circumferences, will be described, and you will use them to determine the BMI, waist-to-hip ratio, and waist 2 circumference. You will also learn to classify an individual's health risk based on these parameters.

KNOW THESE TERMS & ABBREVIATIONS

- [ ] anthropometric = relating to the measurement of the size and proportions of the human body

- [ ] BMI = body mass index: body weight in kg/height in meters squared ($kg \cdot m^{-2}$)

- [ ] epidemiological studies = studies performed on human populations that attempt to link health effects to a cause; e.g., waist circumference and type 2 diabetes

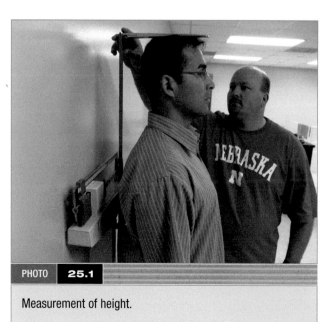

PHOTO **25.1**

Measurement of height.

EQUIPMENT (see Appendix 2 for vendors)	Approximate Price
1. Scale	$175
2. Meter stick	$10
3. Tape measure	$7–$29

PROCEDURES[1,5,6]

1. Measure the subject's height in meters (cm/100) and body weight in kg with the shoes removed (see photos 25.1 and 25.2). Record the values on worksheet 25.1.

2. Identify the landmarks for the waist 1, waist 2, and hips circumferences (see photos 25.3, 25.4, and 25.5).

3. Place the tape parallel to the floor (horizontal).

4. Hold the tape firmly around the circumference site, but do not compress the underlying tissue.

5. Take three measurements per site and use the mean of repeated recordings that agree within 0.5 cm. Record measurements on worksheet 25.1.

Circumference Sites in cm[1,2,6,8]

Waist 1 (see photo 25.3): at the level of the "natural waist," midway between the xyphoid process and umbilicus

Waist 2 (see photo 25.4): at the level of the umbilicus and iliac crests

Hips (see photo 25.5): at the level of the pubis symphysis and the maximal protrusion of the gluteal muscles

Sample Calculations

Gender: _Male_

Body weight: _80 kg_

Height: _1.85 m_

Waist 1: (also called abdomen 1 in Lab 28) circumference: _84.0 cm_

Waist 2: (also called abdomen 2 in Lab 28) circumference: _87.0 cm_

Hips circumference: _96 cm_

body mass index (BMI) = body weight in kg / height in meters squared (kg $\cdot$ m^{-2})

BMI = 80/1.85^2 = 80/3.42 = 23.4

waist-to-hip ratio   = waist 1 circumference in cm / hips circumference in cm

waist-to-hip ratio   = 84.0/96.0 = 0.875

waist 2 circumference   = 87.0 cm

Tables 25.1, 25.2, and 25.3 provide mean height, body weight, and BMI values by age categories.[8]

Tables 25.4, 25.5, and 25.6 provide health risk classifications for BMI, waist-to-hip ratio, and waist 2 circumference.[3,4,5,6,7]

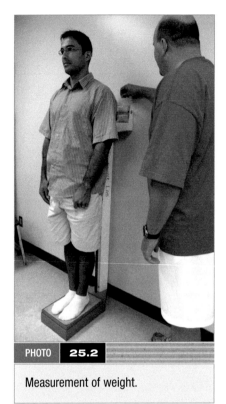

PHOTO   **25.2**

Measurement of weight.

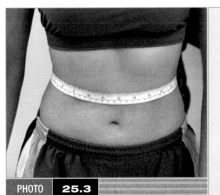

PHOTO   **25.3**

Measurement of waist 1 circumference, at the natural waist.

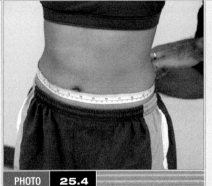

PHOTO   **25.4**

Measurement of waist 2 circumference, at the level of the umbilicus and iliac crests.

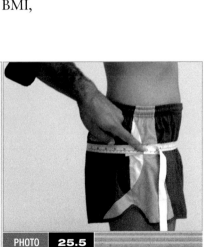

PHOTO   **25.5**

Measurement of hips circumference, at the level of the symphysis pubis and maximal gluteal protrusion.

TABLE	25.1	Mean (± SEM) height (cm) values by age categories.[8]

Age (years)	Males	Females
17	175.3 ± 0.57	163.1 ± 0.56
18	176.4 ± 0.65	163.1 ± 0.44
19	176.7 ± 0.64	162.9 ± 0.64
20–29	176.7 ± 0.29	162.8 ± 0.31
30–39	176.4 ± 0.26	163.1 ± 0.28
40–49	177.2 ± 0.33	163.4 ± 0.24
50–59	175.8 ± 0.32	162.3 ± 0.35
60–69	174.8 ± 0.33	160.6 ± 0.27
70–79	172.7 ± 0.44	159.0 ± 0.31
80 and over	170.7 ± 0.44	155.8 ± 0.34

TABLE	25.2	Mean (± SEM) body weight (kg) values by age categories.[8]

Age (years)	Males	Females
17	75.6 ± 1.38	61.7 ± 1.21
18	75.6 ± 1.12	65.2 ± 1.52
19	78.2 ± 1.29	67.9 ± 1.21
20–29	83.4 ± 0.70	71.1 ± 0.90
30–39	86.0 ± 0.90	74.1 ± 0.91
40–49	89.1 ± 0.73	76.5 ± 1.09
50–59	88.8 ± 0.94	76.9 ± 1.15
60–69	88.2 ± 0.73	76.3 ± 0.76
70–79	82.7 ± 0.71	71.0 ± 0.76
80 and over	76.0 ± 0.66	63.7 ± 1.31

| Mean (± SEM) BMI values by age categories.[8] | | TABLE 25.3 |

Age (years)	Males	Females
17	24.5 ± 0.41	23.1 ± 0.41
18	24.2 ± 0.34	24.4 ± 0.48
19	24.9 ± 0.36	25.5 ± 0.43
20–29	26.6 ± 0.19	26.8 ± 0.29
30–39	27.5 ± 0.26	27.9 ± 0.33
40–49	28.4 ± 0.25	28.6 ± 0.40
50–59	28.7 ± 0.31	29.2 ± 0.40
60–69	28.9 ± 0.20	29.6 ± 0.30
70–79	27.7 ± 0.18	28.0 ± 0.29
80 and over	26.1 ± 0.23	26.1 ± 0.48

| Health risk classifications for BMI.[5] | | TABLE 25.4 |

BMI ($kg \cdot m^{-2}$)	Weight classification	Health risk
<18.5	Underweight	Increased
18.5–24.9	Normal weight	Average
25.0–29.9	Overweight	Increased
≥30	Obese	High

Note: Underweight, overweight, and obese classifications are associated with various diseases such as hypertension, dyslipidemia, and cardiovascular disease.[1]

| TABLE | 25.5 | Health risk classifications for cardiovascular disease associated with waist-to-hip ratio by age categories.[4,6,7] |

Males

Age (years)	Low	Moderate	High	Very High
20–29	<0.83	0.83–0.88	0.89–0.94	>0.94
30–39	<0.84	0.84–0.91	0.92–0.96	>0.96
40–49	<0.88	0.88–0.95	0.96–1.00	>1.00
50–59	<0.90	0.90–0.96	0.97–1.02	>1.02
60–69	<0.91	0.91–0.98	0.99–1.03	>1.03

Females

Age (years)	Low	Moderate	High	Very High
20–29	<0.71	0.71–0.77	0.78–0.82	>0.82
30–39	<0.72	0.72–0.78	0.79–0.84	>0.84
40–49	<0.73	0.73–0.79	0.80–0.87	>0.87
50–59	<0.74	0.74–0.81	0.82–0.88	>0.88
60–69	<0.76	0.76–0.83	0.84–0.90	>0.90

Note: Waist-to-hip ratio uses waist 1 circumference.

| TABLE | 25.6 | Chronic disease classifications for waist 2 circumference.[3] |

Waist 2 Circumference (cm)

Chronic disease risk	Females	Males
Very low	<70	<80
Low	70–89	80–99
High	90–109	100–120
Very high	>110	>120

Note: Chronic diseases include type 2 diabetes, hypertension, and cardiovascular disease.[1]

ANTHROPOMETRIC MEASURES OF HEALTH RISK FORM   Worksheet 25.1

Name _____   Date _____

Gender: ____Male____

Age: ____21____ years

Body Weight: ____~~70.3~~ 65____ kg

Height: ____172.7____ cm / 100 = ____1.72____ meters

	Trial 1	**Trial 2**	**Trial 3**	**Mean**
Waist 1 circumference (cm)	71	72		
Waist 2 circumference (cm)	72	72		
Hips circumference (cm)	72	72		

BMI = body weight in kg / height in m^2 = ____~~70.3~~ 65____ kg / ____1.72____ 2.9 m^2 = ____~~23~~ 22____

Classification = ____normal____ (table 25.4)

Waist-to-hip ratio = waist 1 circumference in cm / hips circumference in cm =

____71____ cm / ____72____ cm = ____0.98____   0.98

Classification = ____High____ (table 25.5)

Waist 2 circumference = ____72____ cm

Classification = ____low____ (table 25.6)

Worksheet 25.2 — EXTENSION ACTIVITIES

Name _____ Date _____

Use the following data and tables 25.4, 25.5, and 25.6 to answer the questions below.

Gender: _____ *female* _____

Age: _____ 20 _____ years

Body weight: _____ 78 _____ kg

Height: _____ 1.75 _____ m

Waist 1 circumference = _____ 82.0 _____ cm

Waist 2 circumference = _____ 89.0 _____ cm

Hips circumference = _____ 98.0 _____ cm

1. Calculate the subject's BMI and classify her health risk (see table 25.4).

   BMI = _____ *(illegible)* _____

   Classification = _____ *Healthy* _____

2. Calculate the subject's waist-to-hip ratio and classify her health risk for cardio-vascular disease (see table 25.5).

   Waist-to-hip ratio = _____

   Classification = _____ *low* _____

3. Based on the subject's waist 2 circumference, classify her health risk for chronic diseases (see table 25.6).

   Classification = _____ *low* _____

EXTENSION QUESTIONS

1. What are some common mistakes that may occur in administering this lab?
2. Identify possible sources of error in this lab.
3. Assess the practicality of using this lab in the field.
4. Research the reliability and/or validity of this lab using the Internet, journal articles, and other credible sources.

REFERENCES

1. American College of Sports Medicine. *ACSM's Guidelines for Exercise Testing and Prescription*, 7th edition, Philadelphia, PA: Lippincott Williams & Wilkins, 2006, pp. 57–61.
2. Behnke, A. R., and Wilmore, J. H. *Evaluation and Regulation of Body Build and Composition*. Englewood Cliffs, NJ: Prentice-Hall, 1974.
3. Bray, G. A. Don't throw the baby out with the bath water. *Am. J. Clin. Nutr.* 79: 347–349, 2004.
4. Bray, G. A., and Gray, D. S. Obesity Part 1—Pathogenesis. *West. J. Med* 149: 429–441, 1988.
5. Expert Panel on the Identification, Evaluation, and Treatment of Overweight in Adults. Clinical guidelines on the identification, evaluation, and treatment of overweight and obesity in adults: Executive summary. *Am. J. Clin. Nutr.* 68: 899–917, 1998.
6. Heyward, V. H., and Stolarczyk, L. M. Applied Body Composition Assessment. Champaign, IL: Human Kinetics, 1996, pp. 81–82.
7. Hoffman, J. *Norms for Fitness, Performance, and Health*. Champaign, IL: Human Kinetics, 2006, p. 87.
8. McDowell, M. A., Fryar, C. D., Hirsch, R., and Ogden, C. L. *Anthropometric Reference Data for Children and Adults: U.S. Population, 1999–2002*. Hyattsville, MD: Centers for Disease Control and Prevention, 2005.

Anthropometric Estimation of Thigh Muscle Cross-Sectional Area

BACKGROUND

The quantification of muscle cross-sectional area (CSA) has been used clinically to evaluate the nutritional status of children, the elderly, and individuals with muscle-wasting diseases or injuries.[3] In nonclinical settings, the quantification of muscle CSA has been used to describe and compare athletic and non-athletic populations, predict muscular strength and strength per unit of muscle CSA, and examine the effects of various interventions on hypertrophy and atrophy.[3]

The most common laboratory techniques used to determine muscle CSA are computed tomography (CT scan) and magnetic resonance imaging (MRI), which are valid and reliable but also expensive (see figures 26.1 and 26.2). Many laboratories do not have access to this technology and, therefore, must rely on more practical methods, such as anthropometry, for assessing muscle CSA. Recently, multiple regression equations for estimating thigh muscle CSA have been developed based on the measurement of the anterior thigh skinfold and mid-thigh circumference.[3] The accuracy (validated against MRI) of these equations is comparable to that of skinfold estimates of percent body fat as well as field tests such as the Astrand–Rhyming test (see Lab 5) for estimating maximal oxygen consumption rate ($\dot{V}O_2$max).[3] The equations are applicable to both males and females. The mid-thigh circumference reflects all tissues of the thigh, including muscle, skin, subcutaneous fat, bone, connective tissue, and vessels. Theoretically, the skinfold accounts for the amount of subcutaneous fat (and skin) that covers the muscle.

In this laboratory, the mid-thigh circumference and anterior thigh skinfold will be measured and used in multiple regression equations to estimate the quadriceps CSA, hamstring CSA, and total thigh muscle CSA. The quadriceps CSA includes the vastus intermedius, vastus lateralis, vastus medialis, and rectus femoris muscles. The hamstring CSA includes the semimembranosus, semitendinosus, and biceps femoris muscles. The total thigh muscle CSA includes the quadriceps, hamstrings, adductor longus, adductor magnus, gracilis, and sartorius muscles.

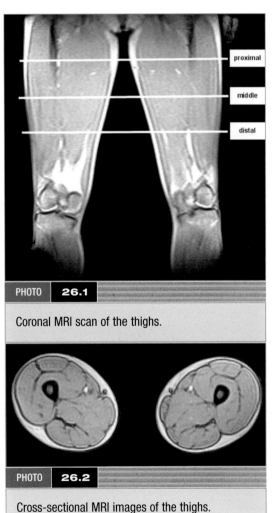

PHOTO **26.1**

Coronal MRI scan of the thighs.

PHOTO **26.2**

Cross-sectional MRI images of the thighs.

KNOW THESE TERMS & ABBREVIATIONS

- ☐ anthropometry = the measurement of the size and proportions of the human body
- ☐ CSA = cross-sectional area. Muscle CSA in this lab is determined using circumferences, skinfolds, and multiple regression equations.
- ☐ CT scan = computed tomography scan
- ☐ MRI = magnetic resonance imaging

- [ ] multiple regression equation = a combination of a number of measurements (independent variables) that best predict a common variable (the dependent variable, in this case muscle CSA)
- [ ] R = multiple correlation coefficient, a numerical measure of how well a dependent variable can be predicted from a combination of independent variables (a number between −1 and 1)
- [ ] SEE = standard error of estimate, a measure of the accuracy of predictions made using a regression equation

EQUIPMENT (see Appendix 2 for vendors)   Approximate Price

1. Tape measure $7–$29
2. Skinfold calipers $150–$480

PROCEDURES

1. Measure and mark the anatomical sites with a marker (see sites below). The mid-thigh circumference and anterior thigh skinfold measurements are taken on the dominant limb. To determine the dominant limb, ask the subject, "Which leg do you prefer to kick with?"
2. Calculate quadriceps CSA, hamstrings CSA, and total thigh muscle CSA using worksheet 26.1. The CSA values from the equations are expressed in cm^2.

Skinfold Site[2]

Anterior Thigh (see photos 26.1–26.3): a vertical fold (measured in mm) on the anterior aspect of the thigh, midway between the hip (inguinal fold) and knee joints (photo 26.1; superior border of the patella).

a. Grasp the skinfold firmly with the thumb and forefinger and pull away from the body (photo 26.2).
b. Hold the caliper perpendicular to the skinfold (photo 26.3). The caliper should be approximately 1 cm away from the thumb and forefinger so that the pressure of the caliper will not be affected.
c. Read the skinfold size approximately one to two seconds after the caliper thumb grip has been released.

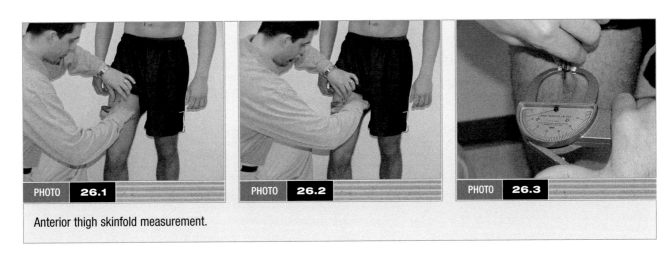

PHOTO **26.1**   PHOTO **26.2**   PHOTO **26.3**

Anterior thigh skinfold measurement.

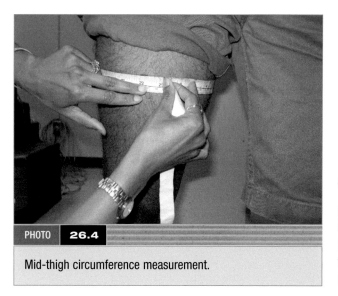

PHOTO   **26.4**

Mid-thigh circumference measurement.

d. Take three measurements (record the measurements on worksheet 26.1) at least 15 seconds apart to allow the skinfold site to return to normal. If the repeated measurements vary by more than 1 mm, more measurements should be taken. Use the mean of the recorded measurements that are within 1 mm as the representative skinfold value in the equations.

Circumference Site[1]

Mid-thigh (see photo 26.4): the distance (expressed in cm) around the thigh, midway between the hip (inguinal fold) and knee joints (superior border of the patella), with the subject standing and feet slightly apart.

a. Place the tape perpendicular to the long axis of the limb.

b. Hold the tape tightly around the limb, but do not compress the underlying tissue.

c. Take three measurements (record the measurements on worksheet 26.1) and use the mean of repeated recordings that agree within 0.5 cm.

Equations[3]

Quadriceps CSA (cm²) = (2.52 × mid-thigh circumference in cm) − (1.25 × anterior thigh skinfold in mm) − 45.13

   R = 0.86

   SEE = 5.2 cm²

Hamstrings CSA (cm²) = (1.08 × mid-thigh circumference in cm) − (0.64 × anterior thigh skinfold in mm) − 22.69

   R = 0.75

   SEE = 3.5 cm²

Total thigh muscle CSA (cm²) = (4.68 × mid-thigh circumference in cm) − (2.09 × anterior thigh skinfold in mm) − 80.99

   R = 0.86

   SEE = 9.5 cm²

Sample Calculations

TRIAL	1	2	3	MEAN
Anterior thigh skinfold (mm)	19.5	20.5	20.0	20
Mid-thigh circumference (cm)	55.0	54.8	55.2	55

Quadriceps CSA (cm²) = (2.52 × 55) − (1.25 × 20) − 45.13 = 68.5 cm²

Hamstrings CSA (cm²) = (1.08 × 55) − (0.64 × 20) − 22.69 = 23.9 cm²

Total thigh muscle CSA (cm²) = (4.68 × 55) − (2.09 × 20) − 80.99 = 134.6 cm²

Table 26.1 includes typical quadriceps, hamstrings, and total thigh muscle
CSA values.

Typical mean (± SD) values for quadriceps, hamstrings, and total thigh muscle cross-sectional area.[3]	TABLE 26.1

Muscle group	Mean ± SD
Quadriceps CSA	75.5 ± 9.9 cm^2
Hamstrings CSA	27.5 ± 5.1 cm^2
Total thigh muscle CSA	145.9 ± 18.3 cm^2

Note: The values listed on this table are for untrained adults (age range = 19–36 years). Training status and age will likely affect the subject's estimated CSA values.

Worksheet 26.1 | ANTHROPOMETRIC ESTIMATION OF THIGH MUSCLE CROSS-SECTIONAL AREA

Name _____   Date _____

Measurements

Trial	1	2	3	Mean
Anterior thigh skinfold (mm)	5	5	_____	_____
Mid-thigh circumference (cm)	5	5	_____	_____

Use the equations on page 180 to calculate:

Quadriceps CSA = _____ cm^2

Hamstrings CSA = _____ cm^2

Total thigh muscle CSA = _____ cm^2

Worksheet 26.2 | EXTENSION ACTIVITIES

Name _____   Date _____

1. A subject's quadriceps CSA estimated from the anthropometric equation in the present laboratory is 70.5 cm^2. Given that the SEE for this equation is 5.2 cm^2, the subject's true quadriceps CSA is likely to fall between what two values?

2. Have your anterior thigh skinfold and mid-thigh circumference measured, and use the anthropometric equations on page 180 to calculate your:

Quadriceps CSA = _____ cm^2

Hamstrings CSA = _____ cm^2

Total thigh muscle CSA = _____ cm^2

EXTENSION QUESTIONS

1. What are some common mistakes that may occur in administering this lab?

2. Identify possible sources of error in this lab.

3. Assess the practicality of using this lab in the field.

4. Research the reliability and/or validity of this lab using the Internet, journal articles, and other credible sources.

REFERENCES

1. Callaway, C. W., Chumlea, W. C., Bouchard, C., Himes, J. H., Lohman, T. G., Martin, A. D., Mitchell, C. D., Mueller, W. H., Roche, A. F., and Seefeldt, V. D. Circumferences. In *Anthropometric Standardization Reference Manual*, eds. T. G. Lohman, A. F. Roche, and R. Martorell. Champaign, IL: Human Kinetics, 1988, pp. 39–54.

2. Harrison, G. G., Buskirk, E. R., Carter, J. E. L., Johnston, F. E., Lohman, T. G., Pollock, M. L., Roche, A. F., and Wilmore, J. Skinfold thicknesses and measurement technique. In *Anthropometric Standardization Reference Manual*, eds. T. G. Lohman, A. F. Roche, and R. Martorell. Champaign, IL: Human Kinetics, 1988, pp. 55–70.

3. Housh, D. J., Housh, T. J., Weir, J. P., Weir, L. L., Johnson, G. O., and Stout, J. R. Anthropometric estimation of thigh muscle cross-sectional area. *Med. Sci. Sports Exerc.* 27: 784–791, 1995.

BACKGROUND

The calculation of an individual's reference weight utilizes diameter measurements (the distance between two bony landmarks) to estimate an appropriate (or normal) body weight based on skeletal size.[1] The reference weight is based on the assumption that diameters and height reflect frame size. In adulthood, frame size provides a stable characteristic from which to estimate how much an individual should weigh with respect to the size of his or her skeleton. The reference weight is the average weight for an adult with a given frame size. Thus, the reference weight can serve as the basis for determining whether an individual is underweight or overweight based on his or her frame size.

The reference weight may also be used in combination with known body composition characteristics (body weight, % fat, fat weight, and fat-free weight) to estimate the changes in fat weight and fat-free weight that are needed to meet a % fat goal at the subject's reference weight. This lab will describe the procedures used to: (1) measure the diameters for the determination of reference weight, (2) calculate the reference weight, and (3) use known body composition characteristics, in conjunction with reference weight, to estimate the changes in fat weight and fat-free weight that are needed to meet a % fat goal at the subject's reference weight.

KNOW THESE TERMS & ABBREVIATIONS

☐ % fat = percent body fat, the proportion of the body that is comprised of adipose (fat) tissue

☐ anthropometer = an instrument used to measure the human trunk and limbs, consisting of two horizontal arms (one movable and one fixed) attached to a vertical rod

☐ fat weight = weight of adipose tissue (subcutaneous and intermuscular and/or intravisceral) and neural tissue

☐ fat-free weight = weight of bone, muscle, tendons, viscera, and connective tissue

☐ reference weight = the average weight for an adult with a given frame size

EQUIPMENT (see Appendix 2 for vendors)	Approximate Price
1. Meter stick	$10
2. Scale	$175
3. Anthropometer	$145–$199

PROCEDURES[1,2]

1. Measure the subject's height in cm and body weight in kg with the shoes removed (see photos 27.1 and 27.2).

2. Palpate for bony landmarks at the diameter sites (see photos 27.4 through 27.11).

3. Hold the anthropometer (see photo 27.3) so that the tips of the index fingers are adjacent to the tips of the blades of the anthropometer.

4. Position the blades of the anthropometer with sufficient pressure to assure that they are measuring bony landmarks.

5. Take three measurements per site and use the mean of repeated recordings that agree within 0.5 cm.

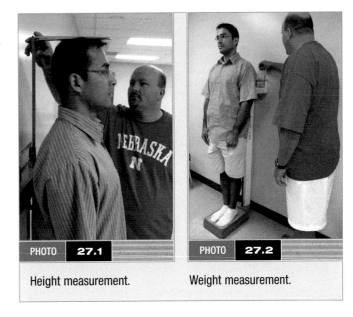

PHOTO **27.1**

Height measurement.

PHOTO **27.2**

Weight measurement.

6. The wrist, elbow, knee, and ankle diameters should be measured on both limbs.

7. Reference weight may be calculated using worksheet 27.1.

Diameter Sites in Centimeters (cm)

Wrist: the distance between the styloid processes of the radius and ulna (see photo 27.4).

Elbow: the distance between the medial and lateral epicondyles of the humerus (see photo 27.5).

Knee: the distance between the medial and lateral epicondyles of the femur (see photo 27.6).

Ankle: the distance between the malleoli (see photo 27.7).

Biacromial: the distance between the most lateral projections of the acromial processes (see photo 27.8).

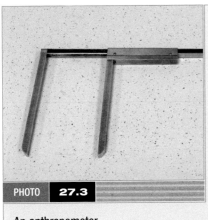

PHOTO **27.3**

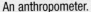

An anthropometer.

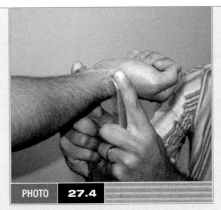

PHOTO **27.4**

Measurement of wrist diameter.

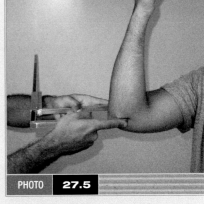

PHOTO **27.5**

Measurement of elbow diameter.

Chest: the distance across the chest at the level of the fifth and sixth ribs (approximately the nipple line) (see photo 27.9).

Bi-iliac: the distance between the most lateral projections of the iliac crests (see photo 27.10).

Bitrochanteric: the distance between the most lateral projections of the greater trochanters (see photo 27.11).

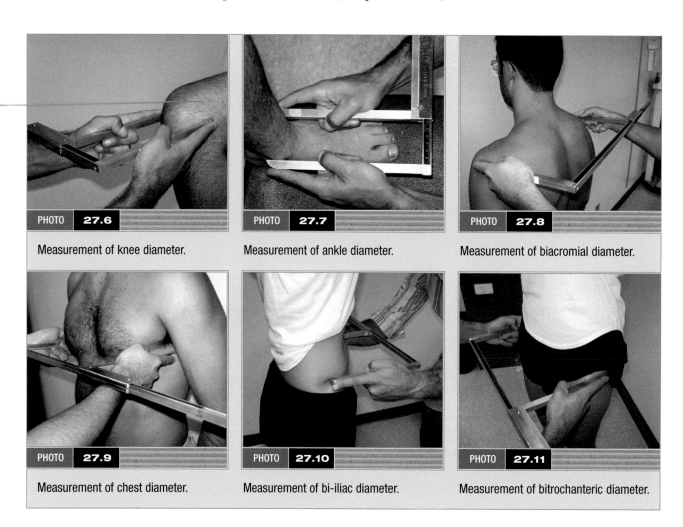

PHOTO **27.6**

Measurement of knee diameter.

PHOTO **27.7**

Measurement of ankle diameter.

PHOTO **27.8**

Measurement of biacromial diameter.

PHOTO **27.9**

Measurement of chest diameter.

PHOTO **27.10**

Measurement of bi-iliac diameter.

PHOTO **27.11**

Measurement of bitrochanteric diameter.

Equation

Sum of diameters = _____ cm

divided by   body constants (31.10 for females, 31.58 for males)   = _____

squared   = _____

times   height (cm)   = _____

times   0.0111 = reference weight   = _____ kg

Body weight (kg) − reference weight (kg) = _____ kg

Classification = _____

Underweight: body weight is at least 5 kg less than reference weight

Normal weight: body weight is within 5 kg of reference weight

Overweight: body weight is at least 5 kg greater than reference weight

Sample Calculations

Height: _176.1 cm_

Body weight: _67.0 kg_

Gender: _Female_

Diameters:

wrist (sum of right and left) = _10.9 cm_

elbow (sum of right and left) = _13.1 cm_

knee (sum of right and left) = _18.0 cm_

ankle (sum of right and left) = _13.3 cm_

biacromial = _34.7 cm_

chest = _24.5 cm_

bi-iliac = _26.9 cm_

bitrochanteric = _31.6 cm_

sum of diameters = _173.0 cm_

	sum of diameters (cm)	= _173.0 cm_
divided by	31.10 (body constant for female)	= _5.563_
squared	5.563 × 5.563	= _30.94_
times	height (cm) = 30.94 × 176.1	= _5449.2_
times	0.0111 × 5449.2 = reference weight	= _60.5 kg_

Body weight minus reference weight = _6.5_ kg of change

Classification = _overweight_

Current body composition characteristics and reference weight may be combined to estimate the change in fat-free weight and fat weight needed to meet a body composition goal at the reference weight.

EXAMPLE:

Current	Goal	Change (goal – current)
Body weight = 67.0 kg	Reference weight = 60.5 kg	60.5 kg – 67.0 kg = –6.5 kg (loss)
% fat = 30%	Target % fat = 20%	20% fat – 30% fat = –10% fat (loss)
Fat weight = 20.1 kg	Fat weight goal (20% of 60.5 kg) = 12.1 kg	12.1 kg – 20.1 kg = –8.0 kg of fat weight (loss)
Fat-free weight = 46.9 kg	Fat-free weight goal (60.5 kg – 12.1 kg) = 48.4 kg	48.4 kg – 46.9 kg = +1.5 kg of fat-free weight (gain)

Note: A positive (+) change means to increase the variable and a negative (–) change means to decrease the variable. Under some circumstances, the combination of body composition and reference weight can result in a recommendation to lose fat-free weight.

Worksheet 27.1   DETERMINATION OF REFERENCE WEIGHT

Name _____   Date _____

Height: _____ cm

Body weight: _____ kg

Gender: _____ Male _____

DIAMETER (cm)

	Right		Mean	Left		Mean	Sum of means
Wrist	5	5	5	5	5	5	10
Elbow	6	6	6	6	6	6	12
Knee	7	7	7	7	7	7	14
Ankle	7	7	7	7	7	7	14
							50

Biacromial	47	___	___
Chest	30	___	___
Bi-iliac	24.7	___	___
Bitrochanteric	___	___	___

Equation

Sum of diameters = __151.7__ cm

divided by body constants (31.10 for females, 31.58 for males) = __4.8__

squared   = __23.04__

times   height (cm) 172   = __825__

times   0.0111 = reference weight   = __0.05__ kg
                                         0.05

Body weight (kg) – reference weight (kg) = __64.95__ kg
65.

Classification = __normal__

Underweight: body weight is at least 5 kg less than reference weight

Normal weight: body weight is within 5 kg of reference weight

Overweight: body weight is at least 5 kg greater than reference weight

Name _____   Date _____

1. Given the following data, calculate the subject's reference weight.

   Height: _180.0 cm_

   Body weight: _75.0 kg_

   Gender: _male_

   Diameters:

Wrist (sum of right and left)	_11.5 cm_
Elbow (sum of right and left)	_15.0 cm_
Knee (sum of right and left)	_22.0 cm_
Ankle (sum of right and left)	_14.5 cm_
Biacromial	_37.0 cm_
Chest	_27.5 cm_
Bi-iliac	_28.0 cm_
Bitrochanteric	_32.5 cm_
Sum of diameters	_____

   Reference weight (see equation on p. 186) = _____ kg

2. Given the data and reference weight from question 1, calculate the required changes in body weight, fat weight, and fat-free weight if the subject currently has 20% fat and has a goal of 15% fat.

Current	Goal	Change (goal – current)
Body weight = 75.0 kg	Reference weight = _____ kg	_____ kg
% fat = 20%	Target % fat = 15%	_____ %
Fat weight = _____ kg	Fat weight = _____ kg	_____ kg
Fat-free weight = _____ kg	Fat-free weight = _____ kg	_____ kg

3. Have your diameters measured and calculate your reference weight. Based on your reference weight, classify yourself as underweight, normal weight, or overweight.

   Reference weight = _____ kg

   Classification = _____

EXTENSION QUESTIONS

1. What are some common mistakes that may occur in administering this lab?

2. Identify possible sources of error in this lab.

3. Assess the practicality of using this lab in the field.

4. Research the reliability and/or validity of this lab using the Internet, journal articles, and other credible sources.

REFERENCES

1. Behnke, A. R., and Wilmore, J. H. *Evaluation and Regulation of Body Build and Composition.* Englewood Cliffs, NJ: Prentice-Hall, 1974.

2. Wilmore, J. H., Frisancho, R. A., Gordon, C. C., Himes, J. H., Martin, A. D., Martorell, R., and Seefeldt, V. D. Body breadth equipment and measurement techniques. In *Anthropometric Standardization Reference Manual,* eds. T. G. Lohman, A. F. Roche, and R. Martorell. Champaign, IL: Human Kinetics, 1988, pp. 27–38.

BACKGROUND

The Somatogram describes an individual's body build or physique. Specifically, the Somatogram uses circumference measures (the distance around a landmark on the body) to determine the distribution of tissues on the body when compared to that of the average (or "normal") adult male or female.[1] For example, it is likely that a weightlifter would have proportionally larger biceps, forearms, shoulders, calves, and chest than the average person. An obese individual, however, may deviate from average by having larger than normal abdominal, hips, and thigh circumferences, while a person who is chronically underweight would likely have a proportionally small abdomen circumference, but large wrist, knee, and ankle circumferences relative to total body measurements.[1] Thus, the Somatogram characterizes the various segments (limbs and torso) of the body based on what is considered proportional for adults. This is accomplished by dividing circumference measures by "segmental constant" values that represent what is average for each site. Segmental constants differ for males and females, because of their unique body build characteristics.

In this laboratory, you will learn the techniques and landmarks for measuring circumferences and use the circumference measurements to develop a Somatogram. See figure 28.1 for an example.

KNOW THESE TERMS & ABBREVIATIONS

- ☐ circumference = the distance around a landmark on the body
- ☐ segmental constant = a value that represents what is average for each circumference site measured
- ☐ Somatogram = a graphic description of body proportions based on circumference measurements (figure 28.1)

EQUIPMENT (see Appendix 2 for vendors)   **Approximate Price**

Tape measure $7–$29

PROCEDURES[1,2]

1. Identify the anatomical landmarks for each circumference (see photos 28.1 through 28.12).
2. Place the tape perpendicular to the long axis of the limb for the extremity sites or parallel to the floor (horizontal) for the torso sites: shoulder, chest, abdomen 1, abdomen 2, and hips.
3. Record all extremity circumferences (wrist, forearm, flexed arm, thigh, knee, calf, and ankle) for both the left and right limbs.
4. Hold the tape tightly around the circumference site, but do not compress the underlying tissue.

FIGURE 28.1   Example Somatogram.

Name   I. M. Sample   Gender   Female

MEASURE	CIRCUMFERENCES (cm)	FEMALE SEGMENTAL CONSTANT	MALE SEGMENTAL CONSTANT	CIRCUMFERENCE/ SEGMENTAL CONSTANT	PROPORTIONAL SCORE
Wrist	15.20	2.73	2.88	5.568	99
Forearm	23.70	4.15	4.47	5.711	102
Flexed Arm	27.85	4.80	5.29	5.802	103
Shoulder	97.60	17.51	18.47	5.574	99
Chest	83.60	14.85	15.30	5.630	100
Abdomen	70.15	12.90	13.07	5.438	97
Hips	94.10	16.93	15.57	5.558	99
Thigh	55.00	10.03	9.13	5.484	98
Knee	36.30	6.27	6.10	5.789	103
Calf	35.75	6.13	5.97	5.832	104
Ankle	21.45	3.70	3.75	5.797	103
Total Body Circumferences	560.70	100.00	100.00	5.607	

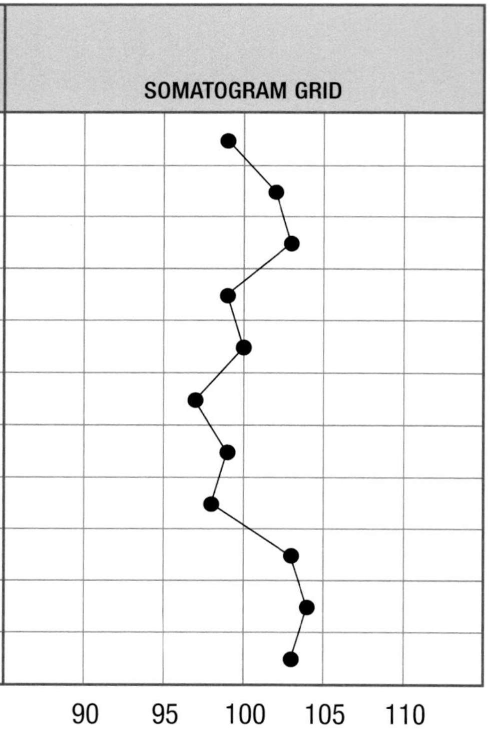

SOMATOGRAM GRID

90   95   100   105   110

5. Take three measurements per site and use the mean of repeated recordings that agree within 0.5 cm.

6. Record on worksheet 28.1 the circumference values for each site. For the extremity sites (wrist, forearm, flexed arm, thigh, knee, calf, and ankle), the circumference value used in the Somatogram is the average of the right and left limbs.

7. Calculate the sum of all circumferences and record it in the box labeled "Total body circumferences." Divide this value by 100 (Total body circumferences/100) and record it in the box directly to the right, under the column "Circumference/segmental constant."

8. Divide each circumference value by the appropriate gender-specific segmental constant and record the values in the boxes to the right under "Circumference/segmental constant."

9. For each circumference, divide the value listed under "Circumference/segmental constant" by the value listed for "Total body circumference/100," then multiply by 100, and record the value in the appropriate box under "Proportional score."

Proportional score = [(Circumference/segmental constant) divided by (Total body circumferences/100)] × 100

10. Plot each proportional score on the adjacent Somatogram grid and connect the points to determine the pattern of the Somatogram.

11. Interpret the Somatogram patterns as follows:

    a. An average body build is indicated when all proportional scores are between 95 and 105.

    b. Body weight versus frame size relationships are reflected in the wrist, knee, and ankle proportional scores. If two or more of these proportional scores are less than 95, overweightness is indicated. If two or more are greater than 105, underweightness is indicated.

    c. Excessive body fat distribution is often reflected in a large proportional score (greater than 105) for the abdomen $\bar{X}$ circumference. Large proportional scores (greater than 105) for the chest, hips, and thigh circumferences may also reflect excessive body fat distributions. The chest and thigh, however, may also be due to extreme muscularity in some males.

    d. Pronounced muscular development is reflected in large proportional scores (greater than 105) for the forearm, flexed arm, shoulders, and calf circumferences.

Circumference Sites in centimeters (cm)

Wrist: the maximal girth (distance around) distal to the styloid processes of the radius and ulna (see photo 28.1).

Forearm: the maximal girth with the arm extended and hand supinated (see photo 28.2).

Flexed arm: the maximal girth over the biceps muscle with the elbow flexed and muscle contracted (see photo 28.3).

Shoulder: across the maximal protrusion of the deltoids (see photo 28.4).

Chest: at the nipple line in males and just above the breast tissue in females (see photos 28.5a and 28.5b).

Abdomen 1 (also called waist 1 in Lab 25): at the level of the "natural waist," midway between the xyphoid process and umbilicus (see photo 28.6).

Abdomen 2 (also called waist 2 in Lab 25): at the level of the umbilicus and iliac crests (see photo 28.7).

Abdomen $\bar{X}$: Average of Abdomen 1 and Abdomen 2 circumferences.

Hips: at the level of the pubis symphysis and the maximal protrusion of the gluteal muscles (see photo 28.8).

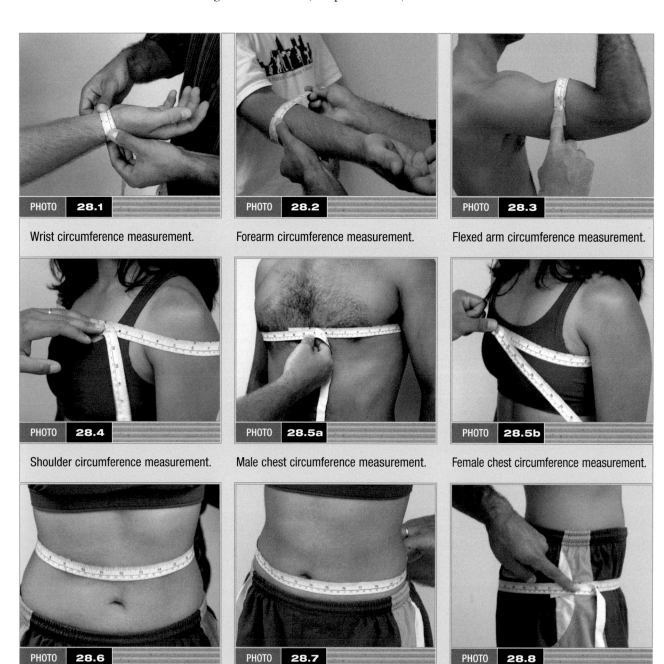

PHOTO **28.1**
Wrist circumference measurement.

PHOTO **28.2**
Forearm circumference measurement.

PHOTO **28.3**
Flexed arm circumference measurement.

PHOTO **28.4**
Shoulder circumference measurement.

PHOTO **28.5a**
Male chest circumference measurement.

PHOTO **28.5b**
Female chest circumference measurement.

PHOTO **28.6**
Abdomen 1 circumference measurement.

PHOTO **28.7**
Abdomen 2 circumference measurement.

PHOTO **28.8**
Hips circumference measurement.

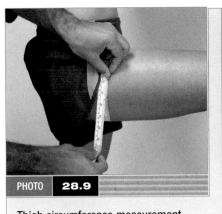

PHOTO 28.9

Thigh circumference measurement.

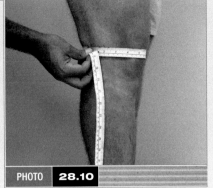

PHOTO 28.10

Knee circumference measurement.

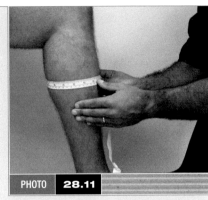

PHOTO 28.11

Calf circumference measurement.

Thigh: the maximal girth inferior to the gluteal fold (see photo 28.9).

Knee: at the level of mid-patella (see photo 28.10).

Calf: the maximal girth (see photo 28.11).

Ankle: the minimal girth superior to the malleoli (see photo 28.12).

Sample Calculations

Figure 28.1 provides a completed sample Somatogram.

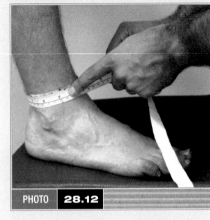

PHOTO 28.12

Ankle circumference measurement.

Worksheet **28.1** SOMATOGRAM

Name _Mohamed. M_

Gender _Male_

Date _10.26.23_

MEASURE	CIRCUMFERENCES (cm)	FEMALE SEGMENTAL CONSTANT	MALE SEGMENTAL CONSTANT	CIRCUMFERENCE/ SEGMENTAL CONSTANT	PROPORTIONAL SCORE	SOMATOGRAM GRID
Wrist	54	2.73	2.88			
Forearm	27cm	4.15	4.47			
Flexed arm	30.3cm	4.80	5.29			
Shoulder	15	17.51	18.47			
Chest	90	14.85	15.30			
Abdomen	247	12.90	13.07			
Hips	34	16.93	15.57			
Thigh	51	10.03	9.13			
Knee	34	6.27	6.10			
Calf	33	6.13	5.97			
Ankle	21	3.70	3.75			
Total Body Circumferences	455	100.00	100.00			

90 95 100 105 110

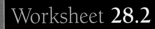

Name _____   Date _____

1. An individual who had proportional scores on the Somatogram of wrist = 90, knee = 93, and ankle = 94 would be classified as (circle one answer below):

    a. Underweight

    b. Overweight

    c. Normal weight

2. An individual with pronounced muscular development would likely exhibit which of the following proportional scores on the Somatogram (circle all correct answers)?

    a. Abdomen $\bar{X}$ = 103

    b. Knee = 92

    c. Flexed arm = 107

    d. Shoulders = 98

    e. Hips = 105

    f. Ankle = 97

    g. Calf = 108

3. Have your circumferences measured, record them on worksheet 28.1, and plot your proportional scores on the Somatogram grid. Based on your Somatogram, classify yourself as underweight, normal weight, or overweight.

    Classification = _____

    What did you base this classification on?

EXTENSION QUESTIONS

1. What are some common mistakes that may occur in administering this lab?

2. Identify possible sources of error in this lab.

3. Assess the practicality of using this lab in the field.

4. Research the reliability and/or validity of this lab using the Internet, journal articles, and other credible sources.

REFERENCES

1. Behnke, A. R., and Wilmore, J. H. *Evaluation and Regulation of Body Build and Composition.* Englewood Cliffs, NJ: Prentice-Hall, 1974.

2. Callaway, C. W., Chumlea, W. C., Bouchard, C., Himes, J. H., Lohman, T. G., Martin, A. D., Mitchell, C. D., Mueller, W. H., Roche, A. F., and Seefeldt, V. D. Circumferences. In *Anthropometric Standardization Reference Manual,* eds. T. G. Lohman, A. F. Roche, and R. Martorell. Champaign, IL: Human Kinetics, 1988, pp. 39–54.

BACKGROUND

Body build characteristics describe an individual's physique.[1,4,5,6] Unlike body composition measurements that determine the relative proportions of fat and fat-free tissue (see Lab 24 on skinfold estimations), body build assessments describe the distribution of body weight on the skeleton.

Athletes in various sports, as well as non-athletes, have unique body build characteristics. For example, basketball players tend to be tall and thin, while football linemen are usually much heavier with a lower center of gravity. Wrestlers and gymnasts, however, tend to be lean and muscular.

In addition to contributing to successful sports performance, body build characteristics can also have health-related implications.[6] For example, the endomorphic rating from the somatotyping procedures in this laboratory has been associated with the risk of developing a number of diseases including coronary heart disease, obesity, and diabetes.[6] Thus, there are both performance and health-related reasons for assessing body build characteristics.

Somatotyping

Somatotyping characterizes body build in terms of the predominance of each of three components: endomorphy, mesomorphy, and ectomorphy. There are a number of ways to perform somatotyping, including the use of photographs (photoscopic method), anthropometry (using height, weight, skinfolds, circumferences, and diameters), or a combination of the two. In this laboratory, the anthropometric method is used to determine the "decimalized anthropometric somatotype."[5,6]

Endomorphy. *Endomorphy,* the first component of the somatotyping classification, rates the individual in terms of fatness or roundness characteristics.

Mesomorphy. *Mesomorphy,* the second somatotype component, describes the individual's muscularity or musculoskeletal development.

Ectomorphy. The third component of the somatotyping classification, *ectomorphy,* rates the individual in terms of linearity of body build based on the relationship between height and weight.

After the separate endomorphy, mesomorphy, and ectomorphy components are calculated, the individual's somatotype characteristics are defined by a three-number combination of the components. That is, an individual who has an endomorphic rating of 2, mesomorphic rating of 3.5, and ectomorphic rating of 5.5 has a somatotype rating of 2-3.5-5.5 (read as 2,3.5,5.5). The first (endomorphy), second (mesomorphy), and third (ectomorphy) components are always listed in the same order. There is no upper limit to the rating scale for each component, but values of 2–2.5 are considered low, 3–5 moderate, 5.5–7 high, and greater than 7.5 very high.[5] Thus, an individual with a somatotype rating of 2-3.5-5.5 has a body build characterized by a low level of fatness (endomorphic rating of 2), moderate muscularity (mesomorphic rating of 3.5), and a high degree of linearity (ectomorphic rating of 5.5). This somatotype rating is typical of a basketball player at the center or forward position.[6] On the other hand, a male body builder may have a somatotype rating of 2-8-1, which reflects a low level of fatness (endomorphic rating of 2), extreme muscularity (mesomorphic rating of 8), and a very low linearity of build (ectomorphic rating of 1).[6] Table 29.1 lists examples of somatotype ratings for non-athletes and athletes in various sports.

TABLE 29.1   Examples of somatotype ratings for non-athletes and athletes in various sports.

Females	Endomorphy	Mesomorphy	Ectomorphy
1. College students[6]	4.2	3.7	2.6
2. Non-athletes[3]	3.57	3.35	2.90
3. Junior Olympic swimmers[14]	3.6	3.4	3.3
4. Professional soccer players[4]	3.07	3.55	2.43
5. Olympic canoers[9]	2.8	4.0	2.9
6. Olympic gymnasts[9]	2.2	3.9	3.4
7. Olympic rowers[9]	3.0	3.9	2.8
8. Olympic swimmers[9]	3.2	3.8	3.1
9. Olympic track & field athletes[9]	2.3	3.4	3.5
10. College basketball players[6]	3.3	3.5	2.8
11. College volleyball players[6]	3.1	3.4	3.2
12. South Australian athletes[17]	3.8	4.2	2.6
13. Body builders[6]	2.5	5.1	2.5
Males	**Endomorphy**	**Mesomorphy**	**Ectomorphy**
1. College students[6]	3.1	5.1	2.7
2. Physical Education majors[7]	2.9	5.4	2.4
3. Young adults 18–29 years[6]	4.1	4.4	2.7
4. Junior Olympic swimmers[14]	2.8	4.5	3.3
5. High school wrestlers[8]	2.77	4.49	3.15
6. South Australian track & field athletes[16]	2.0	4.7	3.4
7. International soccer players[6]	2.5	5.0	2.5
8. Olympic canoers[6]	1.8	5.4	2.6
9. Olympic gymnasts[6]	1.4	5.8	2.5
10. Olympic rowers[6]	2.3	5.0	2.7
11. Olympic swimmers[6]	2.1	5.1	2.8
12. Olympic marathoners[6]	1.4	4.4	3.4
13. Olympic sprinters[6]	1.7	5.2	2.8
14. Olympic basketball players[6]	2.0	4.2	3.5
15. Olympic volleyball players[6]	2.3	4.4	3.4
16. Body builders[6]	1.6	8.7	1.2
17. College football players[6]	4.6	6.3	1.4

KNOW THESE TERMS & ABBREVIATIONS

☐ ectomorphy = the third component of the somatotyping classification, a rating of the individual in terms of linearity of body build based on the relationship between height and weight

☐ endomorphy = the first component of the somatotyping classification, a rating of the individual in terms of fatness or roundness characteristics

☐ mesomorphy = the second somatotype component, a rating of the individual in terms of the individual's muscularity or musculoskeletal development

☐ ponderal index = height in cm / cube root of body weight in kg – a height/weight ratio, estimated either from a nomogram or by use of a calculator

☐ somatochart = a two-dimensional graph on which the X and Y coordinates are calculated from the three somatotype components (endomorphy, mesomorphy, and ectomorphy)

EQUIPMENT
(see Appendix 2 for vendors)

	Approximate Price
1. Meter stick	$10
2. Scale	$175
3. Tape measure	$7–$29
4. Skinfold calipers	$150–$480
5. Anthropometer	$145–$199

Procedures

To calculate the three components of the somatotype rating, 10 anthropometric measurements need to be taken: height, body weight, four skinfolds, two diameters, and two circumferences. The following list includes all of the measurements needed to determine an individual's somatotype rating.

1. Height in centimeters without shoes (inches $\times$ 2.54 = cm; see photo 29.1)

2. Body weight in kilograms without shoes (pounds / 2.2046 = kg; see photo 29.2)

3. Skinfolds in millimeters (inches $\times$ 25.4 = mm)

Procedures to measure skinfolds:

a. Measure and mark the anatomical site with a marker (see sites below).

b. Take all measurements on the right side of the body.

c. Grasp the skinfold firmly with the thumb and finger and pull away from the body.

d. Hold the caliper perpendicular to the skinfold. The caliper should be approximately 1 cm away from the thumb and forefinger so that the pressure of the caliper will not be affected.

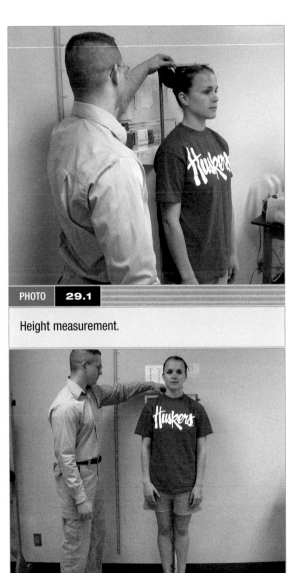

PHOTO **29.1**

Height measurement.

PHOTO **29.2**

Body weight measurement.

e. Read the skinfold size approximately one to two seconds after the caliper thumb grip has been released.

f. Take three measurements per site at least 15 seconds apart to allow the skinfold site to return to normal. Record the skinfold values on worksheet 29.1. If the repeated measurements vary by more than 1 mm, more measurements should be taken. Use the mean of the recorded measurements that agree within 1 mm.

Skinfold Sites[6,10,12]

Triceps: a vertical fold on the posterior midline of the upper arm, halfway between the acromion and olecranon processes; the elbow should be extended and relaxed (see photo 29.3).

Suprailium: a diagonal fold above the crest of the ilium at the spot where an imaginary line would come down from the anterior axillary line (see photo 29.4).

Subscapular: a diagonal fold adjacent to the inferior angle of the scapula (see photo 29.5).

Medial calf: a vertical fold on the medial side of the leg, at the level of maximum circumference of the calf (see photo 29.6).

4. Procedures to measure diameters:
   a. Palpate for bony landmarks of the right limbs (see sites below).
   b. Hold anthropometer so that the tips of the index fingers are adjacent to the tips of the blades of the anthropometer.
   c. Position the blades of the anthropometer with sufficient pressure to assure they are measuring bony landmarks.
   d. Take three measurements per site and use the mean of repeated recordings that agree within 0.5 cm. Record the diameter values on worksheet 29.1.

Diameter sites[6,15]

Elbow: the distance between the medial and lateral epicondyles of the humerus (see photo 29.7).

Knee: the distance between the medial and lateral epicondyles of the femur (see photo 29.8).

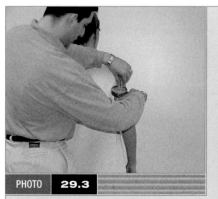

PHOTO **29.3**

Triceps skinfold measurement.

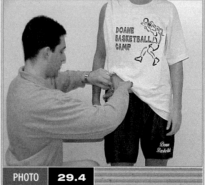

PHOTO **29.4**

Suprailium skinfold measurement.

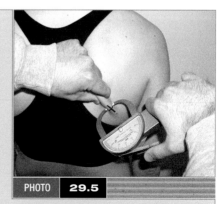

PHOTO **29.5**

Subscapular skinfold measurement.

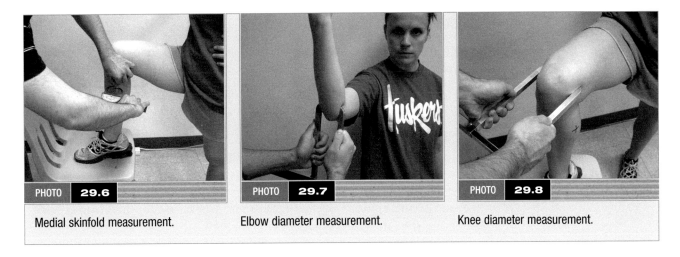

PHOTO 29.6

Medial skinfold measurement.

PHOTO 29.7

Elbow diameter measurement.

PHOTO 29.8

Knee diameter measurement.

5. Procedures to measure circumferences (see photos 29.9–29.10):

   a. Identify the landmarks of the right limbs (see sites below).

   b. Place the tape perpendicular to the long axis of the limb.

   c. Hold the tape tightly around the limb, but do not compress the underlying tissue.

   d. Take three measurements per site and use the mean of repeated recordings that agree within 0.5 cm. Record the circumference values on worksheet 29.1.

Circumference Sites[2,6]

Flexed arm: the maximal distance around the flexed biceps and triceps (see photo 29.9).

Calf: the maximal distance around the calf with the subject standing and feet slightly apart (see photo 29.10).

Equations

The following equations are used to calculate the endomorphic, mesomorphic, and ectomorphic ratings.[5,6]

Endomorphy

Height-corrected endomorphic rating

$= - 0.7182 + 0.1451$ ((sum of triceps, suprailium, and subscapular skinfolds) $\times$ (170.18/height in cm))

$- 0.00068$ (sum of 3 skinfolds $\times$ (170.18/height in cm))^2

$+ 0.0000014$ (sum of 3 skinfolds $\times$ (170.18/height in cm))^3

Mesomorphy

Mesomorphic rating

$= [(0.858 \times$ elbow diameter$) \times (0.601 \times$ knee diameter$) + (0.188 \times$ (flexed arm circumference $-$ triceps skinfold/10))

$+ (0.161 \times$ (calf circumference $-$ calf medial skinfold/10))]

$- (0.131 \times$ height$) + 4.50$

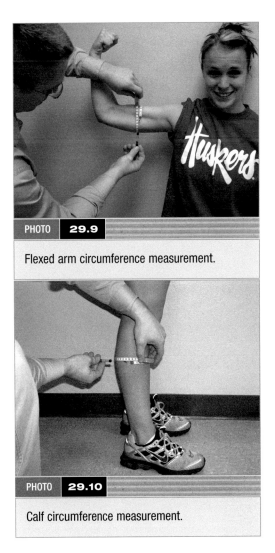

PHOTO 29.9

Flexed arm circumference measurement.

PHOTO 29.10

Calf circumference measurement.

Ectomorphy

The ectomorphic rating is based on the height–body weight ratio or ponderal index.[3,11]

> ponderal index = height in cm/cube root of body weight in kg

The ponderal index can be estimated from the nomogram in figure 29.1. The cube root of body weight can be determined by use of a calculator with a y^x key. To get the cube root, enter body weight, press y^x, enter 0.333, and press "equals."[5]

Based on the ponderal index, the ectomorphic rating is determined as follows:

If the ponderal index is greater than or equal to 40.75, then the ectomorphic rating = 0.732 × ponderal index – 28.58.

If the ponderal index is less than 40.75 and greater than 38.25, then the ectomorphic rating = 0.463 × ponderal index – 17.63.

If the ponderal index is equal to or less than 38.25, then the ectomorphic rating = 0.1.

Sample Calculations

Height: <u>176.0 cm</u>

Body weight: <u>62.8 kg</u>

Triceps skinfold: <u>11.0 mm</u>

Suprailium skinfold: <u>14.0 mm</u>

Subscapular skinfold: <u>9.0 mm</u>

Medial calf skinfold: <u>15.0 mm</u>

Elbow diameter: <u>6.5 cm</u>

Knee diameter: <u>9.0 cm</u>

Flexed arm circumference: <u>27.85 cm</u>

Calf circumference: <u>35.75 cm</u>

Height-corrected endomorphic rating = – 0.7182 + 0.1451 ((11+14+9) × (170.18/176)) – 0.00068 $(32.9)^2$ + 0.0000014 $(32.9)^3$ = 3.36

Mesomorphic rating = [(0.858 × 6.5) + (0.601 × 9.0) + (0.188 × (27.85 – 1.1)) + (0.161 × (35.75 – 1.5))] – (0.131 × 176) + 4.50 = 3.03

Ectomorphic rating

> ponderal index = 176.0/$\sqrt[3]{62.8}$ = 176.0/3.97 = 44.33

Thus, ectomorphic rating = 0.732 × 44.33 – 28.58 = 3.87

Somatotyping rating = 3.36 – 3.03 – 3.87

Somatochart

Somatotype ratings can be visualized and compared to characteristics of various populations by plotting them on a somatochart (figures 29.2–29.4). While the somatotype includes three components (endomorphy, mesomorphy, and ectomorphy), the somatochart plots the somatotype on a two-dimensional graph. To do so, X and Y coordinates are calculated from the three components as follows:[5,13]

Nomogram for determining the ponderal index (height in cm/cube root of weight in kg).   **FIGURE**   **29.1**

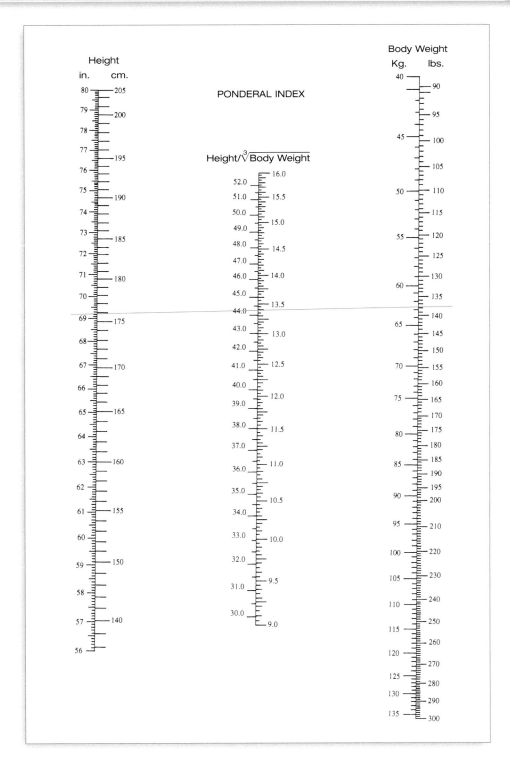

To estimate the ponderal index, lay a ruler between the height on the left column and body weight on the right column. Read the ponderal index value where the ruler crosses the center column. For example, the subject in the sample calculation had a height of 176.0 cm, body weight of 62.8 kg, and a ponderal index of 44.33.

X = ectomorphic rating – endomorphic rating

Y = 2 × mesomorphic rating – (endomorphic + ectomorphic ratings)

The X and Y coordinates can then be plotted on the somatochart. For example, figure 29.2 is the somatochart for the individual with a somatotype of 3.36 (endomorphy)-3.03 (mesomorphy)-3.87 (ectomorphy).

X = 3.87 – 3.36 = 0.51

Y = 2 × 3.03 – (3.36 + 3.87) = –1.17

Figures 29.3 and 29.4 include the somatotypes of various male and female athletes as well as the non-athletes in table 29.1 on somatocharts. Figures 29.5 and 29.6 are blank somatocharts.

FIGURE 29.2 Somatochart for somatotype ratings of 3.36-3.03-3.87 (X coordinate = 0.51 and Y coordinate = –1.17).

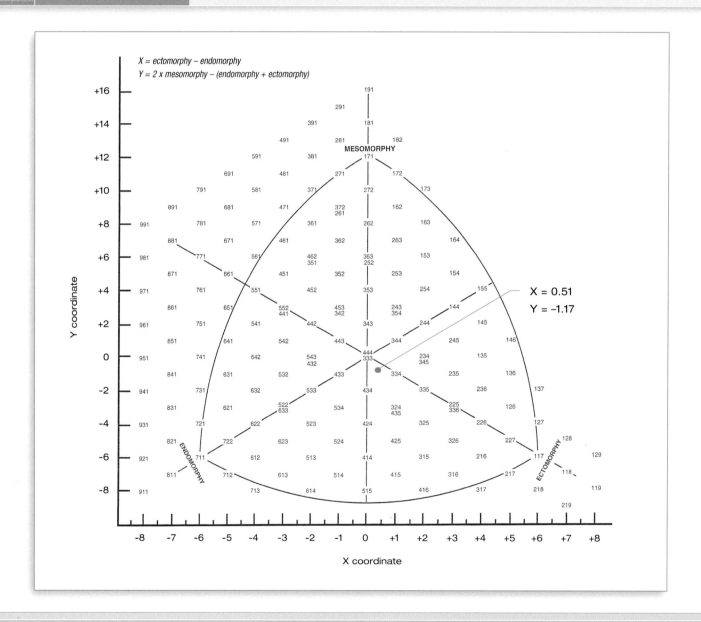

Somatochart examples of male athletes and non-athletes (see table 29.1).   **FIGURE 29.3**

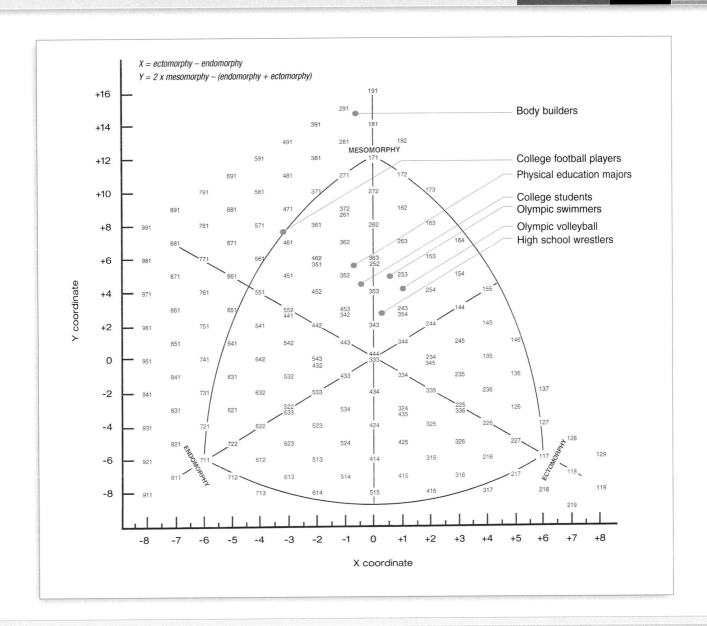

FIGURE   **29.4**   Somatochart examples of female athletes and non-athletes (see table 29.1).

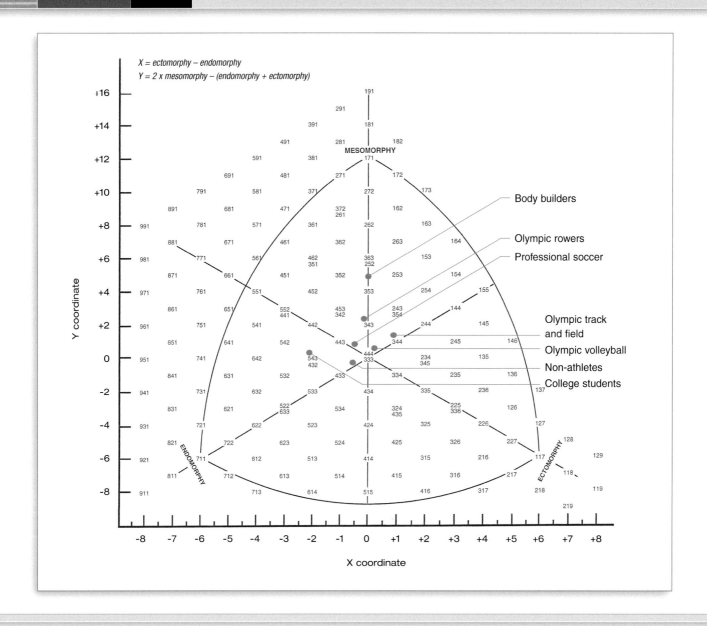

Name _____   *Date* _____

Height: _____ cm

Height-correction = 170.18 / height in cm: _____

Body weight: _____ kg

Trial	**1**	**2**	**3**	**Mean**
Triceps skinfold (mm)	_____	_____	_____	_____
Suprailium skinfold (mm)	_____	_____	_____	_____
Subscapular skinfold (mm)	_____	_____	_____	_____
Sum of triceps, suprailium, and subscapular skinfolds (mm) =				_____
Medial calf skinfold (mm)	_____	_____	_____	_____
Elbow diameter (cm)	_____	_____	_____	_____
Knee diameter (cm)	_____	_____	_____	_____
Flexed arm circumference (cm)	_____	_____	_____	_____
Flexed arm circumference (cm) minus triceps skinfold (mm) / 10 =				_____
Calf circumference	_____	_____	_____	_____
Calf circumference (cm) minus calf skinfold (mm) / 10 =				_____

Endomorphic rating: _____

Mesomorphic rating: _____

Ectomorphic rating: _____

Somatotype rating: _____ – _____ – _____

X coordinate: _____

Y coordinate: _____

Somatochart: Use figure 29.5.

FIGURE   **29.5**   Blank somatochart.

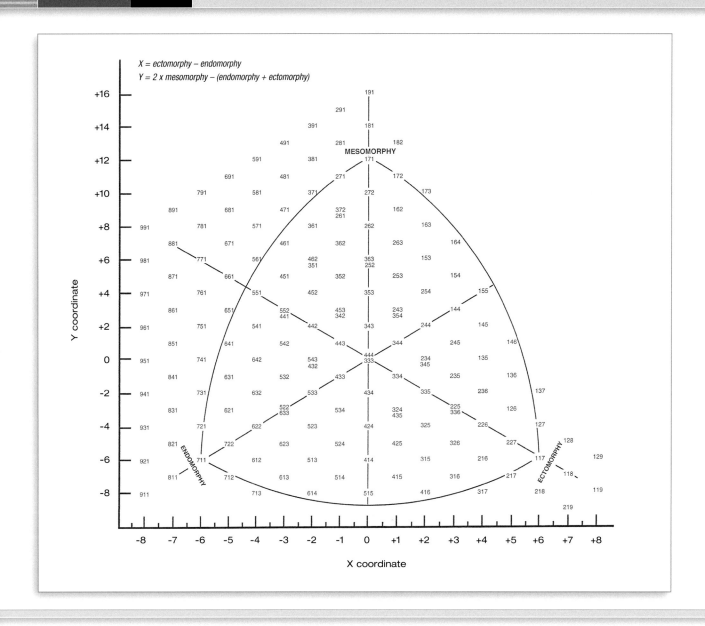

Name _____   *Date* _____

1. Given the following data, calculate: (a) endomorphic rating, (b) mesomorphic rating, (c) ectomorphic rating, (d) X coordinate, and (e) Y coordinate.

    Data:

    Height: _172.0 cm_

    Body weight: _68.5 kg_

    Triceps skinfold: _17.0 mm_

    Suprailium skinfold: _16.0 mm_

    Subscapular skinfold: _13.0 mm_

    Medial calf skinfold: _14.0 mm_

    Elbow diameter: _7.5 cm_

    Knee diameter: _9.0 cm_

    Flexed arm circumference: _29.6 cm_

    Calf circumference: _37.9 cm_

    a. Endomorphic rating: _____

    b. Mesomorphic rating: _____

    c. Ectomorphic rating: _____

    d. X coordinate: _____

    e. Y coordinate: _____

2. Using the somatotype ratings in table 29.1: (a) calculate the X and Y coordinates for female Junior Olympic swimmers; female Olympic canoers; and male Olympic marathoners, and (b) plot these three sets of X and Y coordinates on the blank somatochart in figure 29.6.

	X	Y
Female Junior Olympic swimmers	_____	_____
Female Olympic canoers	_____	_____
Male Olympic marathoners	_____	_____

FIGURE   29.6   Blank somatochart.

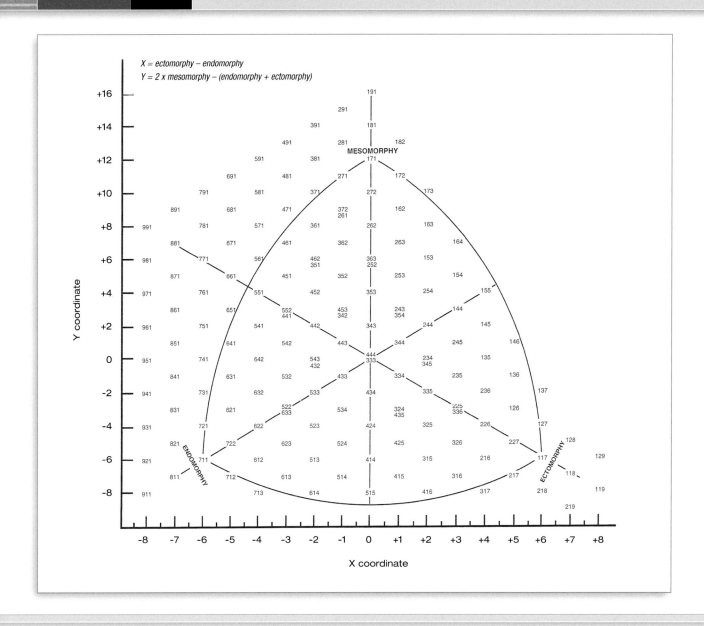

EXTENSION QUESTIONS

1. What are some common mistakes that may occur in administering this lab?

2. Identify possible sources of error in this lab.

3. Assess the practicality of using this lab in the field.

4. Research the reliability and/or validity of this lab using the Internet, journal articles, and other credible sources.

REFERENCES

1. Behnke, A. R., and Wilmore, J. H. *Evaluation and Regulation of Body Build and Composition.* Englewood Cliffs, NJ: Prentice Hall, 1974.

2. Callaway, C. W., Chumlea, W. C., Bouchard, C., Himes, J. H., Lohman, T. G., Martin, A. D., Mitchell, C. D., Mueller, W. H., Roche, A. F., and Seefeldt, V. D. Circumferences. In *Anthropometric Standardization Reference Manual,* eds. T. G. Lohman, A. F. Roche, and R. Martorell. Champaign, IL: Human Kinetics, 1988, pp. 39–54.

3. Can, F., Yilmaz, I., and Erden, Z. Morphological characteristics and performance variables of women soccer players. *J. Strength Cond. Res.* 18: 480–485, 2004.

4. Carter, J. E. L. *The Heath–Carter Somatotype Method.* San Diego, CA: San Diego University Press, 1980.

5. Carter, J. E. L. Somatotyping. In *Anthropometrica,* eds. K. Norton and T. Olds. Sidney, Australia: University of New South Wales Press, 1996, pp. 147–170.

6. Carter, J. E. L., and Heath, B. H. *Somatotyping—Development and Applications.* Cambridge, MA: Cambridge University Press, 1990.

7. Carter, J. E. L., Stepnicka, J., and Clarys, J. P. Somatotypes of male physical education majors in four countries. *Res. Q.* 44: 361–371, 1973.

8. Cisar, C. J., Johnson, G. O., Fry, A. C., Housh, T. J., Hughes, R. A., Ryan, A. J., and Thorland, W. G. Preseason body composition, build, and strength as predictors of high school wrestling success. *J. Appl. Sport Sci. Res.* 1: 66–70, 1987.

9. Cressie, N. A. C., Withers, R. T., and Craig, N. P. The statistical analysis of somatotype data. *Yearbook of Physical Anthropology* 29: 197–208, 1986.

10. Harrison, G. G., Buskirk, E. R., Carter, J. E. L., Johnston, F. E., Lohman, T. G., Pollock, M. L., Roche, A. F., and Wilmore, J. Skinfold thicknesses and measurement techniques. In *Anthropometric Standardization Reference Manual,* eds. T. G. Lohman, A. F. Roche, and R. Martorell. Champaign, IL: Human Kinetics, 1988, pp. 55–70.

11. Housh, T. J., Thorland, W. G., Johnson, G. O., Tharp, G. D., and Cisar, C. J. Anthropometic and body build variables as discriminators of event participation in elite adolescent male track and field athletes. *J. Sports Sci.* 2: 3–11, 1984.

12. Jackson, A. S., and Pollock, M. L. Practical assessment of body composition. *Physician Sportsmed.* 13: 76–90, 1985.

13. Ross, W. D., and Wilson, B. D. A somatotype dispersion index. *Res. Q.* 44: 372–374, 1973.

14. Thorland, W. G., Johnson, G. O., Housh, T. J., and Refsell, M. J. Anthropometric characteristics of elite adolescent competitive swimmers. *Human Biol.* 55: 735–748, 1983.

15. Wilmore, J. H., Frisancho, R. A., Gordon, C. G., Himes, J. H., Martin, A. D., Martorell, R., and Seefeldt, V. D. Body breadth equipment and measurement techniques. In *Anthropometric Standardization Reference Manual,* eds. T. G. Lohman, A. F. Roche, and R. Martorell. Champaign, IL: Human Kinetics, 1988, pp. 27–38.

16. Withers, R. T., Craig, N. P., and Norton, K. I. Somatotypes of South Australian male athletes. *Human Biol.* 58: 337–356, 1986.

17. Withers, R. T., Whittingham, N. O., Norton, K. I., and Dutton, M. Somatotypes of South Australian female games players. *Human Biol.* 59: 575–584, 1987.

Unit 8

FLEXIBILITY

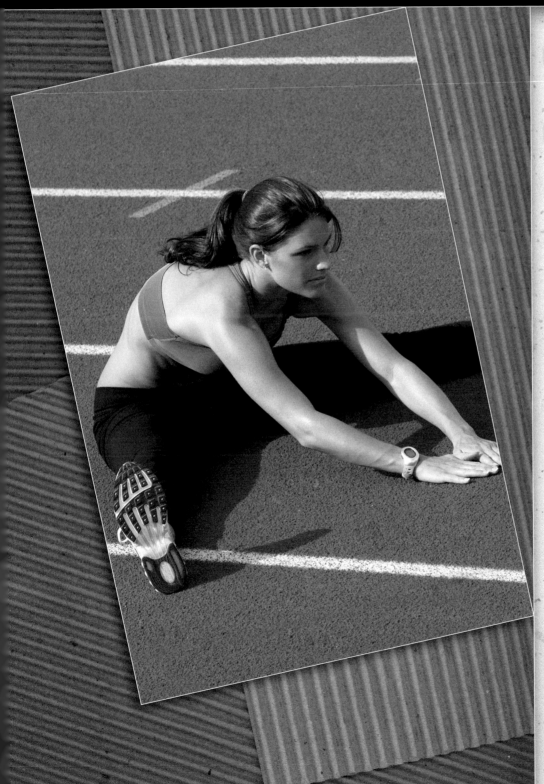

Sit-and-Reach Flexibility

BACKGROUND

Flexibility is a measure of the range of motion at a specific joint. Just because an individual has a large range of motion at the shoulder joint does not mean the person is also "flexible" at the hip joint. Therefore, no single test can adequately represent overall body flexibility. However, many people experience low back pain, which is often related to poor flexibility in the low back and hamstring muscles. Therefore, the sit-and-reach test is the most commonly used measure of flexibility. The sit-and-reach test requires the subject to reach forward, stretching the muscles of the low back and hamstrings. In this laboratory experience, you will learn how to use the sit-and-reach test to evaluate an individual's flexibility, and you will compare the results to norms for individuals of the same age and gender (see tables 30.1 and 30.2).

KNOW THESE TERMS & ABBREVIATIONS

☐ flexibility = a measure of the range of motion at a specific joint

☐ percentile rank = in this lab, a score between 1% and 99% that shows how the subject performed relative to others in the age and gender group. A percentile ranking of 70, for example, indicates that the subject's low back and hamstring muscles are equal to or more flexible than 70% of the others in the age and gender group and less flexible than 30% of the others in the age and gender group.

EQUIPMENT (see Appendix 2 for vendors)   Approximate Price

1. Meter stick $10
2. Sit-and-reach box $117–$275
3. Anthropometer $145–$199

Sample Calculations

Name: _I. M. Flexible_

Gender: _female_

Age: _20 years_

Trial	1	2	3
	20	22	21

High Score = _22_ inches

Approximate percentile rank = _75_ (table 30.1)

Classification = _good_ (table 30.1)

Procedures

1. Have the subject warm up by walking or riding a stationary cycle ergometer and by doing static stretching exercises.

2. Leg position: Have the subject sit down with shoes off with full extension at the knee and feet no more than 8 inches apart. The heels should be at the 15-inch mark on the measuring scale (see note below).

3. Arm position: The arms should be extended straight forward with one hand over the top of the other, fingertips even, and palms down (see photo 30.1).

4. For the test, have the subject reach forward along the measuring scale and hold the position for one or two seconds. Record the point reached on worksheet 30.1, and repeat for a total of three trials.

5. Record on worksheet 30.1 the most distant point reached to the nearest .25 inch. If the fingertips are uneven or if flexion at the knee occurs, the test should be repeated (see photo 30.2).

Note: A sit-and-reach box can easily be constructed. The box should be 12 inches high with an overlap toward the subject so that readings can be obtained if the subject is unable to reach the feet. The foot line is set at 15 inches. A bench (or a floor) with a ruler taped onto it can also be used (see photo 30.3).

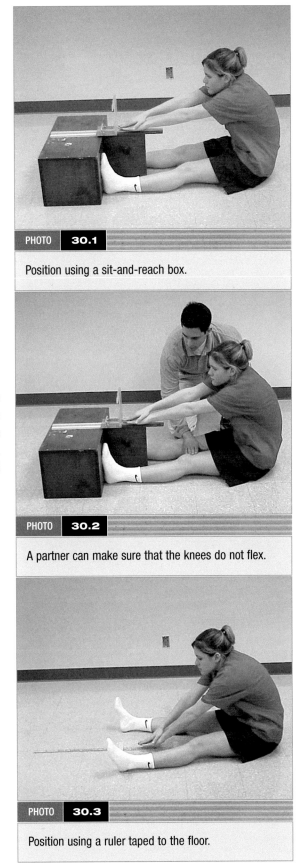

PHOTO **30.1**

Position using a sit-and-reach box.

PHOTO **30.2**

A partner can make sure that the knees do not flex.

PHOTO **30.3**

Position using a ruler taped to the floor.

TABLE   30.1   Percentile norms for the sit-and-reach (in), females.[1]

Percentile	<20	20–29	30–39	40–49	50–59	60+	Classification
99	>24.3	>24.5	>24.0	>22.8	>23.0	>23.0	
95	24.3	24.5	24.0	22.8	23.0	23.0	Superior
90	24.3	23.8	22.5	21.5	21.5	21.8	
85	22.5	23.0	22.0	21.3	21.0	19.5	
80	22.5	22.5	21.5	20.5	20.3	19.0	Excellent
75	22.3	22.0	21.0	20.0	20.0	18.0	
70	22.0	21.5	20.5	19.8	19.3	17.5	
65	21.8	21.0	20.3	19.1	19.0	17.5	
60	21.5	20.5	20.0	19.0	18.5	17.0	Good
55	21.3	20.3	19.5	18.5	18.0	17.0	
50	21.0	20.0	19.0	18.0	17.9	16.4	
45	20.5	19.5	18.5	18.0	17.0	16.1	
40	20.5	19.3	18.3	17.3	16.8	15.5	Fair
35	20.0	19.0	17.8	17.0	16.0	15.2	
30	19.5	18.3	17.3	16.5	15.5	14.4	
25	19.0	17.8	16.8	16.0	15.3	13.6	
20	18.5	17.0	16.5	15.0	14.8	13.0	Poor
15	17.8	16.4	15.5	14.0	14.0	11.5	
10	14.5	15.4	14.4	13.0	13.0	11.5	
5	14.5	14.1	12.0	10.5	12.3	9.2	
1	<14.5	<14.1	<12.0	<10.5	<12.3	<9.2	Very poor

TABLE   30.2   Percentile norms for the sit-and-reach (in), males.[1]

Percentile	<20	20–29	30–39	40–49	50–59	60+	Classification
99	>23.4	>23.0	>22.0	>21.3	>20.5	>20.0	
95	23.4	23.0	22.0	21.3	20.5	20.0	Superior
90	22.6	21.8	21.0	20.0	19.0	19.0	
85	22.4	21.0	20.0	19.3	18.3	18.0	
80	21.7	20.5	19.5	18.5	17.5	17.3	Excellent
75	21.4	20.0	19.0	18.0	17.0	16.5	
70	20.7	19.5	18.5	17.5	16.5	15.5	
65	19.8	19.0	18.0	17.0	16.0	15.0	
60	19.0	18.5	17.5	16.3	15.5	14.5	Good
55	18.7	18.0	17.0	16.0	15.0	14.0	
50	18.0	17.5	16.5	15.3	14.5	13.5	
45	17.3	17.0	16.0	15.0	14.0	13.0	
40	16.5	16.5	15.5	14.3	13.3	12.5	Fair
35	16.0	16.0	15.0	14.0	12.5	12.0	
30	15.5	15.5	14.5	13.3	12.0	11.3	
25	14.1	15.0	13.8	12.5	11.2	10.5	
20	13.2	14.4	13.0	12.0	10.5	10.0	Poor
15	11.9	13.5	12.0	11.0	9.7	9.0	
10	10.5	12.3	11.0	10.0	8.5	8.0	
5	9.4	10.5	9.3	8.3	7.0	5.8	
1	<9.4	<10.5	<9.3	<8.3	<7.0	<5.8	Very poor

SIT-AND-REACH TEST FORM | Worksheet 30.1

Name _Muhamed_   Date _____

Gender _Male_   Age _22_

	Trial 1	**Trial 2**	**Trial 3**
Score (in)	17.5 in	19.2	20.75

High score (in) _20.75_

Percentile rank _~~60~~ 80_

Classification _~~good~~ Excellent_

EXTENSION ACTIVITIES | Worksheet 30.2

Name _____   Date _____

1. Briefly describe the limitation of using a single test of range of motion such as the sit-and-reach test as it relates to overall flexibility.

2. Use your own data from the sit-and-reach test to determine your percentile rank and classification (see tables 30.1 and 30.2). What does your percentile rank mean?

EXTENSION QUESTIONS

1. What are some common mistakes that may occur in administering this lab?
2. Identify possible sources of error in this lab.
3. Assess the practicality of using this lab in the field.
4. Research the reliability and/or validity of this lab using the Internet, journal articles, and other credible sources.

REFERENCE

1. *Physical Fitness Assessments and Norms for Adults and Law Enforcement*, 2007. Cooper Institute, Dallas, TX. Available online at www.cooperinstitute.org.

Lab 31

BACKGROUND

Flexibility is a measure of the range of motion at a specific joint. Just because an individual has a large range of motion at the hip joint does not mean the person is also "flexible" at the shoulder joint. Furthermore, the need for flexibility at a specific joint depends on the sports or activities in which the individual participates. For example, baseball pitchers, gymnasts, swimmers, and wrestlers require great flexibility at the shoulder joint, while swimmers, dancers, divers, and jumpers (long jump, high jump, triple jump, etc.) need substantial ankle flexibility. Therefore, flexibility assessments should be selected based on the demands of the sport or activity.

In this laboratory, you will learn to use the shoulder elevation and trunk extension tests to evaluate an individual's flexibility, and you will compare the results to gender-specific norms for young adults.

KNOW THESE TERMS & ABBREVIATIONS

☐ flexibility = a measure of the range of motion at a specific joint

☐ percentile rank = in this lab, a score between 10% and 90% that shows how the subject performed relative to others in the gender group. A percentile ranking of 70, for example, indicates that the subject's flexibility rating and scores are higher than 70% of the others in the gender group and lower than 30% of the others in the gender group.

☐ static stretching = a stretching method where specified joints are locked into a position that places the muscles and connective tissues passively at their greatest possible length, and held for 10 to 60 seconds

EQUIPMENT (see Appendix 2 for vendors)	Approximate Price
Yardstick	$10

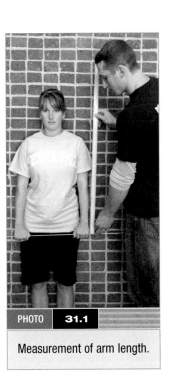

PHOTO 31.1

Measurement of arm length.

PROCEDURES

Shoulder Elevation Test[1,2]

1. The shoulder elevation test requires measuring the subject's arm length, which is defined as the distance between the acromion process (top of the shoulder) and the palm of the hand. To do so, have the subject stand and grasp a yardstick with the arms fully extended and hands pronated (see photo 31.1). Measure the distance (in inches) between the acromion process and the top of the yardstick. Record the arm length on worksheet 31.1.

2. Have the subject warm up by walking or riding a stationary cycle ergometer and doing static stretching exercises of the trunk, shoulders, and arms.

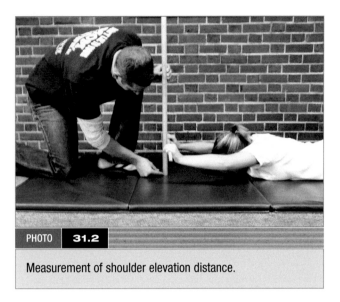

PHOTO **31.2**

Measurement of shoulder elevation distance.

3. Have the subject lie face-down on the floor with the arms fully extended above the head and grasp a yardstick (see photo 31.2). The chin should be touching the floor. Have the subject slowly raise the yardstick from the floor as high as possible. It is important that the subject keep the chin on the floor and arms fully extended while raising the yardstick. Record the distance (in inches) between the yardstick and floor on worksheet 31.1. Repeat for a total of four trials. Use the greatest distance from the four trials in all calculations.

4. Calculate the shoulder elevation score as:

greatest shoulder elevation distance in inches × 100 / arm length in inches

5. Determine the subject's approximate percentile rank and flexibility rating from table 31.1.

Sample Calculations

Gender: _____Male_____

Arm length: _____29 inches_____

Greatest shoulder elevation distance: _____20 inches_____

shoulder elevation score = ___20___ (inches) × 100 / ___29___

= ___2000 / 29___ = ___69 inches___

approximate percentile rank: ___49___ (see table 31.1)

flexibility rating: ___below average___ (see table 31.1)

Trunk Extension Test[1,2]

1. The trunk extension test requires measuring the subject's trunk length, which is defined as the distance between the tip of the nose and the seat

---

TABLE   31.1   Percentile ranks, flexibility ratings, and shoulder elevation scores.[1]

Percentile rank	Rating	Shoulder elevation score (in)	
		MALES	FEMALES
90	Well above average	106–123	105–123
70	Above average	88–105	86–104
50	Average	70–87	68–85
30	Below average	53–69	50–67
10	Well below average	35–52	31–49

of the chair in which the subject is sitting (see photo 31.3). To do so, have the subject sit in a chair, with the back straight and chin level. Place the zero end of a yardstick on the seat of the chair between the subject's legs, and measure the distance between the seat of the chair and the tip of the subject's nose. Record the trunk length on worksheet 31.2.

2. Have the subject warm up by walking or riding a stationary cycle ergometer and doing upper-body static stretching exercises.

3. Have the subject lie face-down on the floor and place the hands on the lower back (see photo 31.4). Have a second person hold down the legs to stabilize the subject. The subject then slowly raises the trunk (hyper-extending the back) from the floor as high and as far back as possible. Record the distance (in inches) between the floor and the tip of the subject's nose on worksheet 31.2. Repeat for a total of four trials. Use the greatest distance from the four trials in all calculations.

4. Calculate the trunk extension score as:

    greatest trunk extension distance in inches × 100 / trunk length in inches

5. Determine the subject's approximate percentile rank and flexibility rating from table 31.2.

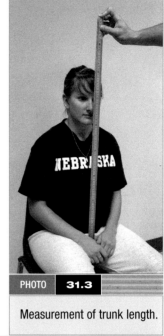

PHOTO   **31.3**

Measurement of trunk length.

Sample Calculations

Gender: ___Female___

Trunk length: ___34 inches___

Greatest trunk extension distance: ___13 inches___

trunk extension score = ___13___ inches × 100 / ___34___

= ___1300 / 34___ = ___38 inches___

approximate percentile rank: ___60___ (see table 31.2)

flexibility rating: ___average___ (see table 31.2)

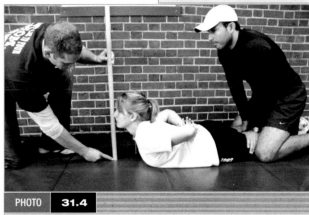

PHOTO   **31.4**

Measurement of trunk extension distance.

Percentile ranks, flexibility ratings, and trunk extension scores.[1]   TABLE   **31.2**

Percentile rank	Rating	Trunk extension score (in)	
		MALES	FEMALES
90	Well above average	50–64	48–63
70	Above average	43–49	42–47
50	Average	37–42	35–41
30	Below average	31–36	29–34
10	Well below average	28–30	23–28

Worksheet **31.1**	**SHOULDER ELEVATION TEST FORM**

Name _____   Date _____

Gender: _____

Arm length: _____ *27* _____ inches

Shoulder elevation distance (inches)

1	2	3	4
16	*16*	_____	_____

Shoulder elevation score = _____ *32* _____

Greatest shoulder elevation distance in inches × 100 / arm length in inches

_____ *96* _____ (inches) × 100 / _____ *27* _____ (inches) = _____ *17* _____ (inches)

Approximate percentile rank: ~~About Average~~ *90* _____ (see table 31.1)

Flexibility rating: _____ *good* _____ (see table 31.1)

Worksheet **31.2**	**TRUNK EXTENSION TEST FORM**

Name _____   Date _____

Gender: _____

Trunk length: _____ *29* _____ inches

Trunk extension distance (inches)

1	2	3	4
~~15~~ *13*	~~15~~ *14*	_____	_____

Trunk extension score = _____

Greatest trunk extension distance in inches × 100 / trunk length in inches

_____ *14* _____ (inches) × 100 / _____ *29* _____ (inches) = _____ (inches)

Approximate percentile rank: _____ *76* _____ (see table 31.2)

Flexibility rating: *Above Average* _____ (see table 31.2)

Name _____   Date _____

1. Use your own data from the shoulder elevation test to determine your approximate percentile rank and flexibility rating (see table 31.1).

    Approximate percentile rank: _____

    Flexibility rating: _____

2. Use your own data from the trunk extension test to determine your approximate percentile rank and flexibility rating (see table 31.2).

    Approximate percentile rank: _____

    Flexibility rating: _____

3. Briefly interpret the meaning of a percentile rank of 50.

4. Identify athletes who might benefit from high shoulder extension and/or trunk extension flexibility.

EXTENSION QUESTIONS

1. What are some common mistakes that may occur in administering this lab?

2. Identify possible sources of error in this lab.

3. Assess the practicality of using this lab in the field.

4. Research the reliability and/or validity of this lab using the Internet, journal articles, and other credible sources.

REFERENCES

1. Acevedo, E. O., and Starks, M. A. *Exercise Testing and Prescription Lab Manual.* Champaign, IL: Human Kinetics, 2003, pp. 76–79.

2. Johnson, B. L., and Nelson, J. K. *Practical Measurements for Evaluation in Physical Education.* Edina, MN: Burgess Publishing, 1986, pp. 91–95.

Distance

1 inch (in) = 2.54 centimeters (cm)

1 foot (ft) = 12 in = 30.48 cm
= 0.3048 meters (m)

1 yard (yd) = 3 ft = 0.9144 m

1 mile (mi) = 5,280 ft
= 1,760 yd
= 1,609.35 m
= 1.61 kilometers (km)

1 m = 39.37 in = 3.28 ft = 1.09 yd

1 km = 0.62 mi

1 m = 100 cm

1 cm = 10 millimeters (mm)

Weights

1 ounce (oz) = 0.0625 pounds (lb)
= 28.35 grams (g)
= 0.029 kilogram (kg)

1 lb = 16 oz = 454 g = 0.454 (kg)

1 g = 0.035 oz = 0.002205 lb

1 kg = 35.27 oz = 2.205 lb

1 kg = 1,000 g

Volume

1 oz = 29.57 milliliters (mL)

1 pint (pt) = 16 oz = 473.1 mL

1 quart (qt) = 32 oz = 2 pt
= 0.9463 liters (L)
= 946.3 mL

1 gallon (gal) = 128 oz = 8 pt = 4 qt
= 3.785 L = 3785.2 mL

1 L = 1,000 mL = 1.057 qt

Energy

1 kilocalorie (kcal) = 1,000 calories (cal)
= 4,184 joules (J)
= 4.184 kilojoules (kJ)

1 L of oxygen (O_2) = 5.05 kcal = 21.139 kJ

1 kilogram meter (kgm) = energy required to move 1 kg 1 m

Power

power = work/time

1 watt (W) = 0.0134 kcal · min^{-1}
= 6.118 kgm · min^{-1}

1 kgm · min^{-1} = 0.1635 W

1 kcal · min^{-1} = 69.78 W

1 MET = 3.5 mL O_2 · kg^{-1} · min^{-1}
= 0.01768 kcal · kg^{-1} · min^{-1}

Velocity

1 mile per hour (mph) = 88 ft · min^{-1}
= 1.47 ft · s^{-1}
= 0.45 m · s^{-1}
= 26.8 m · min^{-1}
= 1.61 kilometers per hour (kph)

1 kph = 16.7 m · min^{-1}
= 0.28 m · s^{-1}
= 0.91 ft · s^{-1}
= 0.62 mph

Temperature

°F (Fahrenheit) = (1.8 × °C) + 32

°C (Celcius, centigrade) = 0.555 × (°F − 32)

°Kelvin = °C + 273

Pressure

1 atmosphere (atm) = 760 mmHg

Equipment	Vendor	Approximate Price
Anthropometer	HOSPEQ, Inc. 7454 SW 48th Street Miami, Florida 33155 (800) 933-0965	$145–199
	Ideal Fitness Inc. P.O. Box 244582 Boynton Beach, Florida 33424 (866) 345-3018	
Anthropometric tape measure	HOSPEQ, Inc. 7454 SW 48th Street Miami, Florida 33155 (800) 933-0965	$12–49
	Power Systems, Inc. 2527 Westcott Blvd. Knoxville, Tennessee 37931 (800) 321-6975	
	Country Technology, Inc. P.O. Box 87 Gays Mills, Wyoming 54631 (608) 735-4718	
Automated sphy-gmomanometer	Country Technology, Inc. P.O. Box 87 Gays Mills, Wyoming 54631 (608) 735-4718	$50–100
	HOSPEQ, Inc. 7454 SW 48th Street Miami, Florida 33155 (800) 933-0965	
Bench press rack	Body Basics 108th & Center in Rockbrook Omaha, Nebraska 68144 (402) 397–8866	$250–500
	Big Fitness 560 Mineral Spring Avenue Pawtucket, Rhode Island 02860 (401) 729–9000	

Equipment	Vendor	Approximate Price
Bench, stair step, or bleacher step (16.25" or 41.3. cm tall)	Power Systems, Inc. 2527 Westcott Blvd. Knoxville, Tennessee 37931 (800) 321-6975	$115
Chalk	Office Discount Club.com 375 Sunrise Highway, Suite 3 Lynbrook, New York 11563 (800) 593-2945	$5
Colored markers *(two or four brightly colored markers, e.g., orange cones, reflective tape, etc.)*	Power Systems, Inc. 2527 Westcott Blvd. Knoxville, Tennessee 37931 (800) 321-6975	$10
	Perform Better 11 Amflex Drive P.O. Box 8090 Cranston, Rhode Island 02920-0090 (800) 556–7464	
Floor mat	Power Systems, Inc. 2527 Westcott Blvd. Knoxville, Tennessee 37931 (800) 321-6975	$20–35
	Perform Better 11 Amflex Drive P.O. Box 8090 Cranston, Rhode Island 02920-0090 (800) 556–7464	
Hand grip dynamometer	Stoelting Corporation 620 Wheat Lane Wood Dale, Illinois 60191 (630) 860–9700	$300
	Johnson Scale 235 Fairfield Avenue West Caldwell, New Jersey 07006 (973) 226-2100	
	Country Technology, Inc. P.O. Box 87 Gays Mills, Wyoming 54631 (608) 735-4718	

Equipment	Vendor	Approximate Price
Heart rate monitor	Polar Electro, Inc. 1111 Marcus Avenue Lake Success, New York 11042-1034 (800) 227-1314 HealthCheck Systems, Inc. 4802 Glenwood Road Brooklyn, New York 11234 (888) 337-4684 Country Technology, Inc. P.O. Box 87 Gays Mills, Wyoming 54631 (608) 735-4718 Perform Better 11 Amflex Drive P.O. Box 8090 Cranston, Rhode Island 02920-0090 (800) 556–7464	$70
Leg press machine	Body Basics 108th & Center in Rockbrook Omaha, Nebraska 68144 (402) 397–8866 Big Fitness 560 Mineral Spring Avenue Pawtucket, Rhode Island 02860 (401) 729–9000	$1,400–1,600
Medicine ball	Perform Better 11 Amflex Drive P.O. Box 8090 Cranston, Rhode Island 02920-0090 (800) 556–7464 Power Systems, Inc. 2527 Westcott Blvd. Knoxville, Tennessee 37931 (800) 321-6975	$29–35
Mercury sphygmo-manometer	Country Technology, Inc. P.O. Box 87 Gays Mills, Wyoming 54631 (608) 735-4718 HOSPEQ, Inc. 7454 SW 48th Street Miami, Florida, 33155 (800) 933-0965	$24–40

Equipment	Vendor	Approximate Price
Meter stick	Science Kit & Boreal Laboratories 777 E Park Dr. Tonawanda, New York 14150 (800) 828-3299 Sargent-Welch PO Box 4130 Buffalo, New York, 14217 (800) 727-4368	$10
Metronome	zZounds Music 65 Greenwood Ave. Midland Park, New Jersey 07432 (800) 996–8637 Sweetwater Sound, Inc. 5501 US Hwy 30 W Fort Wayne, Indiana 46818 (800) 222-4700	$15–16
Monark cycle ergometer	Monark Exercise AB Kroonsvag 1S–780 50 Vansbro, Sweden +46 281 59 49 40 Health Care International Inc. 1723 West Nickerson Street Seattle, Washington 98119 (206) 285-5219 Country Technology, Inc. P.O. Box 87 Gays Mills, Wyoming 54631 (608) 735-4718	$2,000–2,500
Olympic bar	Body Basics 108th & Center in Rockbrook Omaha, Nebraska 68144 (402) 397–8866 Power Systems, Inc. 2527 Westcott Blvd. Knoxville, Tennessee 37931 (800) 321-6975 Perform Better 11 Amflex Drive P.O. Box 8090 Cranston, Rhode Island 02920-0090 (800) 556–7464	$150

Equipment	Vendor	Approximate Price
RPE scale	Young Enterprises, Inc. 25680 Tonganoxie Rd. Leavenworth, Kansas 66048 (800) 765-3975	$18
Scale (eye-level, body weight)	Country Technology, Inc. P.O. Box 87 Gays Mills, Wyoming 54631 (608) 735-4718 HOSPEQ, Inc. 7454 SW 48th Street Miami, Florida 33155 (800) 933-0965 NorthShore Care Supply 3985 Commercial Ave. Northbrook, Illinois 60062 (800) 563-0161	$175–199
Sit-and-reach box (or you can build it)	HOSPEQ, Inc. 7454 SW 48th Street Miami, Florida, 33155 (800) 933-0965 Robbins Sports P.O. Box 2076 Orem, Utah 84059 (866) 754-5355	$117–275
Skinfold calipers	Country Technology, Inc. P.O. Box 87 Gays Mills, Wyoming 54631 (608) 735-4718 HOSPEQ, Inc. 7454 SW 48th Street Miami, Florida 33155 (800) 933-0965 Jansen Medical Supply, LLC 6125 W. Sam Houston Parkway North Suite 201 Houston, Texas 77041-5128 (888) 896-4050	$20–280
Stadiometer	Quick Medical P.O. Box 1052 Snoqualmie, Washington 98065 (888) 345-4858	$13–69

Equipment	Vendor	Approximate Price
Standard Olympic weight plates	Perform Better 11 Amflex Drive P.O. Box 8090 Cranston, Rhode Island 02920-0090 (800) 556-7464 Power Systems, Inc. 2527 Westcott Blvd. Knoxville, Tennessee 37931 (800) 321-6975	$0.69 per pound
Stethoscope	Country Technology, Inc. P.O. Box 87 Gays Mills, Wyoming 54631 (608) 735-4718 HOSPEQ, Inc. 7454 SW 48th Street Miami, Florida 33155 (800) 933-0965	$21–47
Stopwatch	TKO Enterprises, Inc. 220 Etowah Trace Fayetteville, Georgia 30214 (678) 817-5789 Stopwatches USA 118 Bauer Drive Oakland, New Jersey 07436-7046 (800) 771-9112 Country Technology, Inc. P.O. Box 87 Gays Mills, Wyoming 54631 (608) 735-4718	$10
Tape measure	Power Systems, Inc. 2527 Westcott Blvd. Knoxville, Tennessee 37931 (800) 321-6975 Country Technology, Inc. P.O. Box 87 Gays Mills, Wyoming 54631 (608) 735-4718	$7–29

% fat   percent fat, the proportion of the body comprised of adipose (fat) tissue

1 mile   1.6 km

1-RM   one repetition maximum, a standard index to quantify muscle strength, referring to the maximum amount of weight that can be lifted one time

ACSM   American College of Sports Medicine

anthropometer   an instrument used to measure the diameters of the human trunk and limbs; consisting of two horizontal arms (one movable and one fixed) attached to a vertical rod.

anthropometric   relating to the measurement of the size and proportions of the human body

anthropometry   the measurement of the size and proportions of the human body

ARC   anaerobic running capacity (km), the y-intercept of the total distance (TD) versus TL relationship (see figure 12.3b)

ATP   adenosine triphosphate

auscultation   listening to sounds arising from organs to aid in diagnosis and treatment

AWC   anaerobic work capacity (kgm), the y-intercept of the work limit (WL) versus time limit (TL) relationship (see figure 11.2b)

BMI   body mass index; body weight in kg/height in meters squared (kg • m^{-2})

BP   blood pressure, a measurement of the forces of the blood acting against the vessel walls during and between heartbeats, measured in millimeters of mercury (mmHg)

BW   body weight

circumference   the distance around a landmark on the body

correlation coefficient   a numerical measure of the degree to which two variables are linearly related (a number between –1 and 1)

CP   critical power (kgm • min^{-1}), the slope coefficient of the work limit (WL) versus time limit (TL) relationship (see figure 11.2b)

CSA   cross-sectional area

CT scan   computed tomography scan

CV   critical velocity (km • hr^{-1}), the slope coefficient of the total distance (TD) versus TL relationship (see figure 12.3b)

DB   body density

DCER   dynamic constant external resistance

diastolic blood pressure   the pressure recorded between heartbeats (diastole)

ectomorphy   the third component of the somatotyping classification, a rating of the individual in terms of linearity of body build based on the relationship between height and weight

endomorphy   the first component of the somatotyping classification, a rating of the individual in terms of fatness or roundness characteristics

epidemiological studies   studies performed on human populations that attempt to link health effects to a cause, e.g., waist circumference and type 2 diabetes

Fat weight   adipose tissue (subcutaneous and intermuscular and/or intravisceral) and neural tissue, abbreviated FW

Fat-free weight   bone, muscle, tendons, viscera, and connective tissue, abbreviated FFW

fatigue index   a number that reflects the anaerobic fatigue capabilities of the muscles that are active during cycling

flexibility   a measure of the range of motion at a specific joint

hand grip dynamometer   an instrument that measures isometric hand grip strength, providing a simple method for characterizing overall body strength

hip extensors   the gluteal muscles (gluteus maximus and gluteus medius) and the hamstrings (biceps femoris, semitendinosus, and semimembranosus)

HR   heart rate, measured in beats per minute (bpm)

HR monitor   equipment used to measure and monitor heart rate, usually including a chest strap (which identifies the heartbeats and transmits the signal telemetrically) and a digital display (which displays the signal as a real-time HR value)

hyperextend   to extend a joint beyond the normal range of motion

hypertension   an abnormally high BP reading (≥140/90)

isometric strength   tension production by a muscle without movement at the joint or shortening of the muscle fibers

kgm • min^{-1}   kilogram meters per minute

231

Korotkoff sounds sounds emitted as a result of pressure exerted against blood vessel walls, providing the basis of traditional BP assessments

leg extensors the quadriceps, made up of the rectus femoris, vastus lateralis, vastus intermedius, and vastus medialis

maximal effort vertical jump total jump height

mean power the total work performed during the 30-second Wingate test (measured in kgm • 30 sec^{-1}) (see Lab 20)

mesomorphy the second somatotype component, a rating of the individual in terms of muscularity or musculoskeletal development

MRI magnetic resonance imaging

multiple regression equation a combination of a number of measurements (independent variables) that best predict a common variable (the dependent variable)

muscular endurance the ability to perform repeated muscle actions that often utilize the same muscles

muscular strength the maximal force that can be exerted by a specific muscle or muscle group

nomogram a graph that shows the relationship between variables

P power output (measured in kgm • min^{-1} or Watts)

palpation the act of examining by touch

PAR-Q Physical Activity Readiness Questionnaire, a medical screening assessment that determines who may be at risk during exercise

peak power the greatest work performed during any five-second period (measured in kgm • 5 sec^{-1}) of the Wingate test (see Lab 20)

percentile rank a score, expressed as a percentage, that shows how the subject performed relative to others in a specified group. A percentile ranking of 70, for example, indicates that the subject's score is higher than 70% of the others in the group and lower than 30% of the others in the group.

ponderal index a height/weight ratio, estimated either from a nomogram or the use of a calculator, equal to height in cm / cube root of body weight in kg

power (force × distance) / time

PWC$_{HRT}$ physical working capacity at the heart rate threshold (measured in Watts), defined as the y-intercept of the power output versus HR slope coefficient relationship (see figure 13.1b)

PWC$_{RPE}$ physical working capacity at the ratings of perceived exertion threshold (measured in Watts), defined as the y-intercept of the power output versus RPE slope coefficient relationship (see figure 14.2b)

R multiple correlation coefficient, a numerical measure of how well a dependent variable can be predicted from a combination of independent variables (a number between −1 and 1)

recovery heart rate the HR taken after the end of exercise

reference weight the average weight for an adult with a given frame size

regression equation a statistical method developed and used to relate two or more variables

RFWT Rockport Fitness Walking Test

risk stratification categorization of the likelihood of untoward events based on the screening and evaluation of patient health characteristics

RPE ratings of perceived exertion

SEE standard error of estimate, a measure of the accuracy of predictions made using a regression equation

segmental constant a value that represents what is average for each circumference site measured

Somatochart a two-dimensional graph on which the X and Y coordinates are calculated from the three somatotype components (endomorphy, mesomorphy, and ectomorphy)

Somatogram a graphic description of body proportions based on circumference measurements

speed the ability to cover a specific distance as fast as possible

sphygmomanometer the instrument used to measure blood pressure in an artery, consisting of a pressure gauge and a rubber cuff and used with a stethoscope. Mercury and aneroid sphygmomanometers are available.

static stretching a stretching method where specified joints are locked into a position that places the muscles and connective tissues passively at their greatest possible length and held for 10 to 60 seconds

systolic blood pressure the pressure exerted against the vessels during a heartbeat (systole)

TL time limit or time to exhaustion (min)

total body power a combination of upper- and lower-body power [(force × distance) / time] output

V̇O$_2$ oxygen consumption rate, an indirect measure of aerobic energy production

V̇O$_2$ max maximal oxygen consumption rate

V̇CO$_2$ the volume of CO_2 produced

v velocity (km • hr^{-1})

VT ventilatory threshold, an estimation of the exercise intensity above which anaerobic ATP production must supplement aerobic metabolism

W Watts

WanT Wingate Anaerobic Test

WL Work limit or total work performed (kgm)